BODYSENSE

The Hazard-Free Fitness Program
for Men and Women

BODYSENSE

The Hazard-Free Fitness Program for Men and Women

Sue Luby

Richard A. St. Onge, M.D.

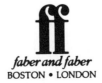

faber and faber
BOSTON • LONDON

Published by
Faber and Faber, Inc.
50 Cross Street
Winchester, MA 01890

Printed in the United States of America

Library of Congress Cataloging-in-Publication Data
Luby, Sue, 1938-
   Bodysense, the hazard-free fitness program for men and women.

   1. Exercise. 2. Posture. 3. Joints—Range of motion. 4. Physical fitness. I. St. Onge, Richard A. II. Title.
   RA781.L83   1986   613.7'1   85-27460
   ISBN 0-571-12546-8 (pbk.)

Sue Luby, owner and operator of the Body Control Center in Andover, Massachusetts for the past eighteen years, offers on-site lodging and workshop vacations at her new Bodysense Training Center in New Hampshire. As a fitness consultant, she has designed conditioning programs for football and track teams and created personal fitness regimens for members of the Boston Bruins hockey team. She is an advisor to Sports Medicine Resources and works with doctors to augment their treatment programs. Sue often travels to give workshops and lectures and has appeared on television several times. A frequent contributor to newspapers and magazines, this is her third book. For additional instructional material for individual and group study programs, which includes video tapes and posters, write:
Sue Luby's Bodysense Training Center
Province Road
Barrington, NH 03825

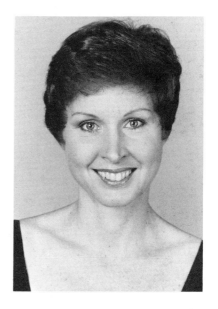

Richard A. St. Onge, M.D. is an orthopaedic and hand surgeon and medical director of Sports Medicine Merrimack Valley in Haverhill, Massachusetts. He is also affiliated with Sports Medicine Resources in Boston. A frequent author of journal articles, he is also a contributor to *Sports Health: The Complete Book of Athletic Injuries* by William Southmayd, M.D. and Marshall Hoffman. An avid participant in many sports, he has been a climber and expedition doctor to the American Club Himalayan Expeditions for three years. Recently, he was a member of the first successful American team climb on Mount Himal Chuli. He lives in Massachusetts.

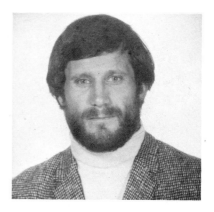

Dedicated to my students who are the source of my education and inspiration. Their enthusiasm for the Bodysense Method has encouraged me to formalize the process in book form.

I especially remember the students from my workshop circuits around the country who, because we cannot maintain routine contact, expressed the desire for hands-on guidance for their own personal regimens and teachings.

I hope this book fulfills their need.

Table of Contents

Foreword

Why write another exercise book? Today, 57 million Americans of all ages are finding fitness to be a rewarding and healthful part of their lives and, in many instances, a necessary part of thriving in a stress-filled world. We see evidence of this interest in exercise all around us: on TV, in the proliferation of health clubs, and in the workplace where enthusiasts often take a jogging lunch. Newsstands, bookstores, and libraries now abound with periodicals devoted to exercise and activity. *Why* then is Sue Luby's Bodysense Method new or different or even necessary in this environment where the message seems to be shouting at us from all sides? Don't we all know how to run, jump, stretch, and exercise? Unfortunately, we don't, especially without causing painful and debilitating injuries to ourselves.

In the 1950s and 1960s, a change came about in the consciousness of American's fitness psyche. Exercise became better understood and was emphasized as an important part of all our lives. It was not just restricted to stereotypes of jocks and athletes running around in sweaty gymnasiums. Exercise and fitness were touted nationally by the President's Council on Fitness, and school programs emphasized fitness at the grassroots levels. Marathon running started to attract media attention, and people, in general, became more interested in sports, such as tennis and racquetball. The once-obscure sports soon had easily recognizable superstars.

Happily, Americans have now accepted the idea of exercise and fitness as being beneficial to their health. The problem is not instructing people *to* exercise, but rather instructing them *how* to exercise. If you exercise improperly or with improper equipment, you are defeating the very purpose for which you exercise. This can result in pains, strains, and injuries that may not only affect your sports, but your daily work as well. Injuries that occur as the result of individuals, regularly active or inactive, participating in exercise and recreational endeavors are what I call *diseases of activity*.

The human body is made to perform athletically. The heart, lungs, muscles, tendons, ligaments, and bones are strengthened and a general sense of well-being and euphoria is created by routine exercise. However, it is clear that exercise performed repetitively and in an improper fashion can stretch ligaments, tear muscles, and fracture bones, which causes pain, disability, disappointment, and depression. No sport or exercise is entirely free from injury. The message today is not to exercise but to *exercise properly*.

No longer is it sufficient for people to bounce a few times on their toes, bend over, touch the ground, and tear off for a seven-mile run. No longer is it acceptable for people to buy a mat, place it on the floor and do repetitive sit-ups. No longer is it considered helpful for people to brace their leg on the back of a car, bend forward with their chin to their knee, and take off down the road in a sprint. These and many other standard and frequently seen stretching techniques are becoming recognized as the causes and not the prevention of problems and injuries. No longer is it suitable for people to sit in cars and behind desks all week and then charge off on weekends to the tennis court and play vigorous sets. No longer is it reasonable to ask the body of any individual after many years of relative physical inactivity to suddenly jump into an aerobics class and try to keep pace with the instructor.

Professional athletes, who know and depend upon their bodies for performance and their careers, spend many years developing and training their bodies' reflexes, strengths, and flexibility. More and more professional athletes realize that a full-time, year-round physical fitness program is necessary for performing at an optimal level. They are participating in stretching/flexibility courses not only before practices or games but on a routine daily basis as well. No professional football player would think of merely putting on the pads and going to play in the Super Bowl without years of training and preparation. Yet, everyday I see men and women decide they are going to take up exercise; go to a health club, YMCA, or their local park, bounce up and down a few times in a half-hearted attempt to stretch; and take off down the road. Increasingly, I see these same individuals coming to sports medicine clinics and doctor's offices with torn Achilles' tendons and hamstrings, tight groins, aching backs, shin splints, and even stress fractures.

My personal encounter with athletically related injuries began when I played football and wrestled in high school and college. I suffered many injuries during those years. Most were minor strains, pulls, and contusions but some were severe knee injuries and ligamentous disruptions, torn shoulder muscles, and fractures. I have had multiple surgeries on both knees and on my back. I sometimes think that there is hardly a patient who has come to me with a problem that I haven't experienced at one time or other. Like many of them, I am still active in sports. I enjoy canoe racing, white-water kayaking, rock and ice climbing, and mountaineering. I utilize running, bicycling, cross-country skiing, and weight lifting as training techniques to maintain fitness for these sports.

My experience with Sue Luby goes back about eight years when, as an orthopaedist and sports medicine specialist, I questioned some of the dogma and routine exercise regimens that I was taught both in my medical and athletic training. At the same time, many more of my patients were presenting me with problems related to sports and activity, which stimulated further questioning of the current exercise programs. Increasingly, my practice was composed of individuals, male and female of all ages, who had problems not of disease but of *injuries of activity*—related directly to their desire and willingness to participate in athletic activities and exercise routines. I struggled from my own experience in training and with the difficulties of my patients to find ways to lessen the effects of the injuries and prevent their recurrence. I began to review the fundamentals of anatomy and physiology, which every doctor learns and studies in medical school. I started to look again at such things as the stretch reflex, which is the spinal column's response of muscles to contract when they are stretched rapidly. This response is subconscious and uncontrolled. I realized that many of the stretches we have been taught to use in the old days asked us to bounce and stretch. This is entirely contrary to the stretch reflex physiology. Instead of achieving the gradual stretch of a muscle or joint, this practice results in a tightness and rebound and can actually tear and injure the muscle. This kind of ballistic stretching is now well-recognized as harmful and, fortunately, is no longer taught by coaches and trainers. However, this is only one example of exercise practice that we grew up thinking was correct and helpful, which actually works to the contrary.

Similarly, many studies have shown that the sit-ups we endlessly did—and sadly, many still do—to strengthen our abdominal muscles and to lose weight are harmful when performed in the standard fashion. The abdominal muscles are critical to the continued strength and endurance to help support the lower back. No doubt, you are familiar with the everyday terms used to designate strength and courage, such as "guts" or "intestinal fortitude." It is often true, that such clichés reflect reality—in this case, it is particularly true.

My search for alternative ways to exercise led me to investigate Bodysense. I had heard of Sue Luby; she was a fitness instructor in a nearby community and had developed an excellent reputation both from her students and other instructors. I approached her with many questions: What is it you do? How do you do it? Does it work? *Why* does it work? I asked her to show me and explain what she did and why she believed in it. At first, I was not convinced—I was even a bit skeptical. Her techniques seemed sound, and her explanations were good and well-reasoned. However, what really assured me was watching her. Her alignment, control, flexibility, and vitality were obvious. The more I watched her and tried the techniques myself, the more convinced I became that she had found something of value.

The importance of Bodysense is that, for the first time, you are shown *what you are doing wrong,* in addition to the correct way to exercise. Bodysense emphasizes, in a carefully selected and detailed way, how important it is to be flexible and teaches the techniques to gain and maintain flexibility. Special attention is given to illustrating and describing *why* and *how* so many of

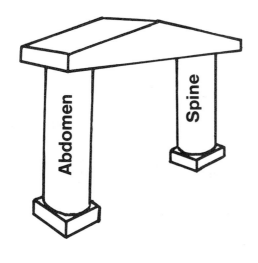

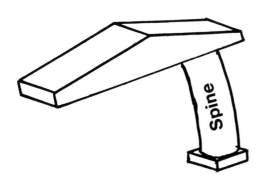

the common stretches and exercises we see used—and we ourselves use—are wrong and hazardous. Bodysense can be useful to everyone to help transmit good intentions in exercising into good practice. It can allow all of us to understand better the mechanics and benefits of using proper, simple, and basic techniques, such as breathing, postural alignment, joint and muscle control, stretching, and flexibility. Athletes, professional and recreational, from the elite to the ordinary enthusiast to those who suffer from multiple musculo-skeletal problems, such as low back pain, flat feet, and knock-knees, have benefitted from Bodysense.

One of the Bodysense principles is alignment. To realize how important this is, picture the spine. It is comprised of a series of block-like bones called vertebral bodies, which are, in the erect posture, piled one on another in a gently arching vertical column. The ligaments and powerful short acting muscles support and control the motion of the spine, which in turn supports the entire body. The spine, however, is located at the back of the body, while a lot of weight, in the form of the chest and abdomen, is located in the front. This imbalance is exaggerated further when a heavy load is carried in front of the body, as we normally carry loads with our hands. Extra and crucial support is needed for the front of the body as well as for the back. This is how the abdominal muscles come into play and how they contribute to the strength and health of the back.

Think of a two-column support system for a platform with a weight or a roof on top of it. Together, the front and back columns can easily support the weight; but if the front column were removed, the back column would be stressed excessively into a bending position and would fall. This is similar to what happens in the body when the back (spine, muscles, and ligaments) is required to solely support the body in all its work functions. The vertebral bodies and disc material between them are compressed and tilted, the ligaments are stressed, and the muscles are strained. In time or with extra loads, the back system fails, bringing pain, spasm, and dysfunction. Everyone has felt this at one time or another.

With strong and flat active abdominal muscles, however, the anterior or front column is strong and useful to support the back and prevent an overload on the spine and discs. The abdominals also contribute strength and stability to the back by controlling the position of the pelvis, which is the foundation on which the back and torso is maintained. If the abdominal muscles are weak and inactive, the lower spine arches excessively into "lordosis" or forward curve. This position adds extra compression, stress, and strain to the vertebral bodies, ligaments, and muscles. When the abdominal muscles are strong and active, they help draw up the pelvis and make it more horizontal, thereby decreasing the excessive curvature of the lower spine. The result is a better balanced and aligned spine that is stronger, more functional, and less painful.

To strengthen the abdominal muscles, which can alleviate lower back problems, sit-up exercises are often prescribed. The goal is laudible but, unfortunately, most of the time sit-ups are done wrong, which not only cannot increase abdominal strength but, even worse, can lead to increased back stress and pain. Doing sit-ups and abdominal exercises improperly can actually increase your back pain problem.

How can this happen? A study of muscle activity (measured by electromyography) and spine flexion (measured by X-ray) was conducted a few years ago at Stanford University. The standard full sit-up exercise of lying flat with the legs flat or lying flat with the hips and knees bent and coming to a full sit-up position was tested against the partial sit-up of lying flat with the hips and knees bent but with only the head and shoulder blades raised off the floor. When all the data was reviewed, it was found that 60 percent of the effort of the sit-up was not performed by the abdominal muscles (rectus abdominus and external obliques) in the full sit-up, but 95 percent of the sit-up activity in the partial sit-up (raising the head and shoulder blades off the floor) was performed by the abdominal muscles. This study demonstrates that the standard full sit-up with the legs either straight or bent and coming to a full upright position cannot strengthen the abdominal muscles because these muscles are not involved primarily in achieving this position. To strengthen the abdominal muscles, one must raise only the head and shoulder blades off the floor, hold it, then slowly return to the floor, and repeat the cycle.

An additional study further verified the adverse effects of the full sit-up position. Lateral X-rays were taken of the lower back in a full sit-up position and showed that the spine was bent forward so much that it caused compression in flexion of the spine and discs and stress and strain on the ligaments posteriorly in the back. Measurement studies revealed that this compression in flexion of the spine is significant. It increases the pressure on the discs and eventually can lead to degenerative changes of the discs and even disc rupture. While not primarily utilizing the abdominals, the action of the full sit-up falls on the deep back muscles called the ilio psoas, which are attached to the spine and pass along to the front of the hip. When these muscles strive to pull the body to a full upright position, they actually cause strain in the lower back as well as a tightening of the hips. A sit-up performed in this fashion definitely is harmful to the back, and excessive and persistent sit-ups practiced in this fashion can only lead to increased back pain and problems.

When only a modified or partial head and shoulder raise sit-up is performed, the spine remains nearly in its normal curvatures in the lower back without excessive compression pressures on either the spine or the discs. Practicing this sit-up, therefore, protects the spine against excessive pressures and, at the same time, strengthens the primary abdominal muscles.

Not only can you adapt the Bodysense Method to correctly

practice your everday exercises, such as sit-ups, you can improve your running performance as well. Running certainly is one of the most natural exercises you can do. The human body is well-designed to run. It exercises your heart as well as the large lower leg muscles. It can be maintained continuously for long periods of time and on a frequently repeated basis. Almost everyone can run. Today, there are perhaps as many as thirty million runners of all ages in America and over seventy thousand who run at least one marathon a year.

For myself, like many others, running is not only healthful physically, but emotionally as well. Runners experience a sense of well-being and sometimes an elation associated with their running. They often become addicted to their daily running routines and feel cheated or less than well when they miss their running session. Scientists have now discovered evidence of human hormones (called endorphines) that are released during the running activity. These occur naturally and are very similar to the opiates used in medicine and probably can be called our internal "pain killers." This may explain why so often the minor discomforts and stresses of the running effort gradually give way to the sensation of comfort and relaxation during a run.

While running is natural, healthful, and relaxing and can help you maintain fitness, cope with stress, and sleep better, it can also cause pain, injury, and disability. Repetitive motion of running in a measured stride for long distances tends to create tight fascia in the feet, tight tendons in the back of the calf and hamstrings, and tightness around the pelvis and lower back. Gradually, tendinitis and inflammation of these areas become prominent. Today, there may be as many as forty million running-related injuries a year. Most are minor sprains and strains, but some become chronic. All interfere with the runner's ability to continue running and to enjoy it.

Clearly, it seemed to me that runners needed a good daily stretching program. It was with these patients that Sue Luby and I started in our initial cooperative effort. I began to send her a few select running patients who were becoming tight and disabled. The results of the Bodysense program were astonishing! Runners not only improved but also decreased the incidences of their tendinitis and strains. In addition, they gradually regained and even increased their flexibility that had been lost for years. They felt better, ran better, and had fewer injuries. This was fascinating and positive evidence of the effectiveness of the Bodysense program.

I remember one patient especially well. He was an ultra-marathon runner at the elite level with a couple of fifty- and seventy-five-kilometer national championships to his credit. Nonetheless, for over a year before I had seen him, he had struggled and was plagued by pain and inflammation in his hips, groin, and back—which was in spasm. His hamstrings and groin muscles were tight and contracted, and his knees and heels were tender and inflamed. He was running sideways like a crab. After the initial period of rest and treatment with anti-inflammatory medicines, we began a routine of gradual, progressive, dynamic stretching on a twice-a-day basis, founded on Sue Luby's Bodysense Method. In far less time than he had already missed because of his injuries, he began to improve. In a dramatic example of the interrelatedness of flexibility to performance, his running returned to its former style and level, as his hamstrings, Achilles' tendons, and groin and back muscles increased their flexibility. He was delighted with the results, and I had greater interest in the Bodysense techniques.

After the experience with the runners, I began to think that some of the nonathletic and nonactive patients could also benefit from a structurally precise stretching, breathing, and body-alignment program, as in Bodysense. The patients who seemed to need rehabilitation the most with this technique were the ones with back pain suffered from mechanical causes (not neurological deficits). They had low back pain; tight hamstrings; excessive lordosis; weak, flabby abdominal muscles; and were generally overweight. These sufferers are quite common, for back pain is universal. Everyone and anyone can get back pain sometime in their lives. For many, it is a constant pain and frustration; for some, it is a crippling disability. Back pain has been recognized as the plague of mankind. The early Egyptians, five thousand years ago, recognized it as a major problem. Today, back pain affects at least one-half of the working population and annually counts for billions of dollars in lost wages and expenses.

It was with these back-pain patients that Sue Luby and the Bodysense stretching techniques impressed me most. Sue's careful technique, clear instructions, intuitive insight and refreshing, enthusiastic approach helped most, if not all, of the patients I sent to her. She developed useful props to help them correct their postures, improve their alignment, and work on their flexibility. Again, most of these patients were not runners or athletic but were all comers, male and female, of all ages, sizes, and shapes. Most were out of shape and did not have a clear understanding of body alignment or exercise. Some had never even used their bodies in exercise.

I recall one woman who came to me with many years of low back pain. She was a skillful business woman and a hard worker but rarely exercised. She spent most of her time riding in automobiles between sales calls and appointments. Progressively, she developed disabling pain not only in her back but also down one of her legs. When I saw her, surgery had been recommended. She was in pain and was fearful and frustrated. After the initial rest and anti-inflammatory medical treatment, her leg pain disappeared; but her back pain continued. I then put her on a gradual and careful rehabilitative program with Sue and Bodysense.

Six months later, this woman was feeling much better than she had felt in many years. She was stretching and swimming daily and enjoying her exercise. She was free from back pain and functioned with more energy and more optimism than she had

had in a long time. She was a delighted patient and a triumph. She was also a very clear example of how useful the correct method of exercise and stretching can be. She commented near the end of her treament, as many others have since, that she wished she had found out "how to stretch and exercise sooner!"

These were the people who demonstrated that Sue Luby's Bodysense program has application for almost everyone. When I saw runners learn how to stretch properly and increase their training times and distances with fewer injuries, I was convinced. When I saw middle-aged and even elderly men and women afflicted with long-standing back pain, who had not been physically active, respond to Sue and her techniques, come back excited, and exclaim that they never felt better, their pain was gone, and they felt more energized, I was moved and convinced.

Our program of collaboration has widened to include other patients, such as young scoliosis patients. These are usually adolescents, boys and girls, who have a curvature of the spine because of bony abnormalities in the development of the spine. As these patients began to stretch daily and to loosen and elongate their spines and supporting ligaments and muscles (especially utilizing Sue's careful instruction about the control of the pelvis and stretching the hamstrings), they began to minimize the negative effects of their spinal abnormalities and increase their flexibility. When this program was combined with a spinal bracing program, the patients did better than I had ever seen such patients do before and were enthusiastic about their treatment.

So, why the necessity of another exercise book? *Bodysense* is the first book to clearly outline the hazards of improper exercise and stretching and to demonstrate specific techniques for correct positive and dynamic stretching and alignment that is so important and that is the basis of all activity and performance in exercise. It can teach people from many backgrounds and all ages to exercise efficiently, effectively, and safely. The Bodysense principles and techniques succeed not because Bodysense is another form of exercise, but because it is a *process* that develops and enhances your *own* flexibility, alignment, and control to prepare your body for movement and performance. It is a rational and careful method of rehabilitation from and prevention of injuries. You will be able to exercise and participate in your sports and everyday activites more energetically and safely.

Remember, health is more than the absence of disease. It is the positive state of existence that encourages active participation in living, physically as well as emotionally. Good health based on exercise creates a sense of well-being and gives reserve energy not only to perform your everyday activities but to respond creatively to the extra demands and stresses as well. Exercising correctly in a hazard-free method enhances health and happiness and improves life—and that's what exercising with Bodysense is all about!

Richard A. St. Onge, M.D.
October 1985

Acknowledgments

I greatly esteem the input and personal experience of B. K. S. Iyengar's work, which was imparted to me through his long-time students and my personal teachers, Dona Holleman, Ramanand Patel, and Judith Lasaters. Their patience and expertise have increased the depth of my awareness and understanding of the great living machine—the human body.

My special thanks go to Fran McCormick and Ruth Williams, my two associates, who now have been a team through all three of my books. Fran diligently worked and reworked her sensitive illustrations to meet both of our professional standards. Ruth's expertise in photography is augmented by her knowledge of Yoga, both as a student and teacher.

Nancy Wilson has my appreciation for her ingenuity, superb writing skills, and tireless assistance.

Thank you to Karen Kozlowski, a fellow Yoga teacher, for her support, helpful critique, and final reading of the manuscript.

I am grateful to Louise Richardson, editor, for having the insight and initiative to take on the big Bodysense project. Her persistence and dedication in seeing that this book is done properly is most appreciated.

My sincere appreciation and love go to my husband, Ralph, for his limitless patience; skillful assistance in building my Fitness Centers; and continual encouragement for me to develop, refine, and teach my Bodysense message.

Dick St. Onge has been of invaluable assistance. He helped organize the manuscript and reviewed the text and artwork for medical accuracy. I can't say enough about his support and firm belief in my work. This gave me the encouragement to continue to create the Bodysense Method. I look forward to our future collaboration in the sports medicine world—Here's to Bodysense fitness!

Sue Luby
December 1985

Section I

Introduction to Bodysense:
The Hazard-Free Fitness Program
for Men and Women

1. Overview

The human body is a living machine working for us under the best and worst of conditions—many of the latter are brought on by our habits. Most of us take our bodies for granted. We neglect them for long periods of time, then press them to their limits when playing sports or when starting an exercise program. We push our bodies despite warning signs of pain, fatigue, and shortness of breath. We do not know our bodies, their limitations and their possibilities.

I am dedicated to teaching people to know their bodies better. I wrote this book to help people dramatically improve performances in sports; develop sound work habits; and foster total well-being in their minds, bodies, and spirits. I want to reach the sports world, physical education teachers, and others who deal with the human body, by showing a wholly different exercise method. I also want to reach those who are just not comfortable in their bodies.

Daily at my Body Control Center, I see athletes, weekend jocks, and regular exercise buffs who hurt themselves because they diligently exercise without knowing their personal alignment patterns and body limitations. The problems are twofold: doing incorrect exercises and doing correct exercises incorrectly.

Doctors such as orthopaedic surgeon Richard A. St. Onge are seeing more and more people suffering from sports injuries because the athletes are not conditioning properly. Many runners who relate their back pain to running should consider the way they are doing their stretching exercises before they run; the way they hold their bodies in everyday life and during sports; and the vigorous, repetitious movements involved in some sports that overwork one side of the body to the detriment of the other. Sports are fine, but many people doing sports have anatomical irregularities to begin with that show up under the strain of sports. A valid conditioning program can balance the misalignments and compensate for the one-sidedness of a particular sport.

When I go into gyms and health clubs, I see men with rounded shoulders use a weight machine and do fifty lifts that tend to round the shoulders and three lifts that tend to open the chest. The lifts that open the chest are hard for them to do and, hence, are not as pleasing psychologically; so they don't do many. But what they don't know is that the pleasing lifts are reinforcing all the negative patterns about their bodies: rounding their shoulders, collapsing their lungs, curtailing their breathing. What they need is somebody to show them how to open their bodies to oxygen, work with alignment, and exercise for health.

I think the human body is designed to run, do yoga, and play tennis—all those things—if they are done with balance. So that's what I'm about: freeing people and helping them to become more efficient so their bodies turn on. Then they can do whatever they want to do.

In contrast to other exercise programs, Bodysense is a Method and does not aim directly at muscular development with an imposition of strength from without. Instead, Bodysense develops strength from within. With caution and an anatomical background, my students come to understand their body patterns and work with consideration of them; they never force the body into positions that are unnatural. That is not to say they pamper their misalignments, but they work on correcting them gradually, without sudden or violent moves.

I learned the importance of alignment the hard way. I came to study Yoga for the same reason that so many of my students now come to me. I was tense, nervous, overweight, and had a pot belly and back problems. The Yoga classes helped me a lot, but there was a time when I felt I wasn't getting far. My back was actually becoming aggravated. Ultimately, I was left to my own devices to work out my problems. I thought that something had to be missing in the execution of the exercises. I then dedicated myself to finding out how *my* unique body worked and how each part of the body was supposed to work. Through studying anatomy and kinesiology, I found out I had cross-eyed knees and one leg shorter than the other. These deficiencies, along with my other problems, had to be factored into my exercise program.

I embarked on applying the principles of alignment to all my body movements. I started putting the exercises under a microscope and insisting that each be executed with the body acting as a single unit that is balanced and controlled. Through my twenty years of study and teaching, I evolved my own approach called Bodysense and discovered it worked. My body grew stronger and healthier. I shared my method and saw others responding positively—even dramatically—to my approach

The pain of my experience made me particularly sensitive to the needs of beginners. I saw so many students who couldn't touch their toes. I started to identify "what parts needed oiling" and then devised ways to awaken and develop those parts properly. To this day, the lessons of my students expand the horizons of Bodysense. I could see my motto, "You control your body; don't let it control you," come to life. Medical doctors, psychiatrists, psychologists, and athletic coaches have enthusiastically endorsed my method because of its preventive and therapeutic nature.

The alignment, stretching, strengthening, and relaxation gained from this program helps to assuage any strain incurred by sports, ballistic, or momentum-type exercises. Whatever the sport, Bodysense helps during the warm-up, play, and post-game slowdown.

Anyone can gain from Bodysense: the athlete who needs to

learn how to move in sports and the nonathlete who needs to learn how to be more comfortable with his or her body.

Too many exercise programs leave people drained and tired. They are boring to do and, because of that, they encourage sloppiness. With no pleasure in the doing plus exhaustion and stiffness to look forward to at the end, people miss a day and then stop bothering entirely.

Through working with Bodysense, you will find that boredom and exhaustion don't have to be anymore. My goal is mental and physical harmony and rejuvenation. No day is exactly like any other, of course, and on some days you'll feel like exercising less than on others; but once you have some experience with the Bodysense Method, you'll come to look forward to the stimulation it can provide. And as time passes, you will also find that, without conscious effort, you are walking and sitting straighter and moving more gracefully. Your muscles will become firmer and sleeker, better shaped, and stronger without being large and bulky. You will be more supple, calmer, and relaxed and be able to enjoy the sport or activity you love—with a new sense of control and inner harmony.

People will comment on how good you look. Your clothes will fit better. You won't have those daytime energy dips. A familiar chair will feel different, because you are sitting straighter. One day, you'll realize it's easier to reach for something you've dropped in an awkward corner under your desk; another day, you'll catch a glimpse of yourself in a mirror or shop window and be surprised at how straight you are standing without seeming forced or stiff.

How does Bodysense bring about these changes? In a surprisingly simple way, as you will see!

2. Before You Begin

Who Can Use This Book

Bodysense can be practiced by everybody with beneficial results.

Adults, who work away from or at home, can adapt this program to their schedules and attire. Many people perform portions of Bodysense by pausing for a few relaxing breaths and correct stretches.

Youngsters and teenagers derive benefits from Bodysense, such as attaining coordination and motor skills in a non-competitive setting. For the child who doesn't play team sports, individual achievement can help develop poise and a good self-image. For all children, the breathing and flexibility techniques are good warm-ups for any physical activity including competitive sports.

Expectant mothers can have better circulation and fewer leg and back complaints, in addition to having a body that is better prepared for delivery, when they practice the Bodysense Method during pregnancy.

All the reasons for practicing Bodysense apply doubly to senior citizens. Relaxation and good breathing can help make the later years more pleasant; for as flexibility and circulation improve, the body becomes rejuvenated and the mind more alert. Age itself is not a limiting factor. I have students who are eighty-years old. Remember—you are as young as your spine is supple.

Bodysense can help you discover and correct weaknesses and imbalances you have and ones you never knew you had; thus, it's possible to overcome present injuries and prevent future ones. Let's see if you are a candidate for future injuries. Do take the Hazards and Personalized Total Fitness Tests (section II).

See Your Doctor

Always check with your doctor before embarking on this, or any, exercise program, and then proceed gently.

When people come to my Body Control Center (Some of them are sent by their physicians.), I custom-design programs of exercise for them based on their individual conditions. In this book, I present a general program and remind you not to do anything that brings on strain or pain. I also strongly recommend that you show this book to your doctor so that he or she will know how you will be exercising. Your doctor is best qualified to diagnose potential problems. This conference is especially important if you have been sedentary, little more than a weekend jock, or are over forty.

Read the Instructions

Before you begin to do the exercise, read the procedures and check your alignment of the particular body area so that you will have a good understanding of the Bodysense Method. Although you may notice some repetition in explanations or instructions, all the information applies to each exercise; so read the instructions thoroughly—they are important in their entirety. Don't just skim and depend on the figures with their directive arrows.

What's in This Book

You will be able to easily understand and learn to use the Bodysense Method through the visual presentation and my teaching tips, which are based on the conditions I saw on 90 percent of my students. As you use the program, you will develop a physical sensitivity to and increasing awareness of the correct way your body should function. Soon it will become part of your nature.

In section II, chapter 1, you will take a test on the sixteen most commonly practiced exercises and check off the ones you think are good to do. I will then discuss each exercise.

In section II, chapter 2, I will give you a test that will let you experience just how flexible you are and what kind of balance you have. This probably will be a different type of fitness test than you have ever taken before, which should prove an enlightening challenge.

Section III, chapter 1 is on breathing, the most important function for our bodies; yet we take it for granted. You will learn the correct way to breathe—don't just laugh it off, thinking you're alive and well and your breathing just automatically works. By applying proper breathing techniques, you can relax, increase your capacity and stamina, and ease the strain that occurs when playing a sport or exercising.

Posture is the subject for section III, chapter 2. This is the second most important factor to good health habits and one that is always overlooked. If your posture is not aligned, you will eventually run into problems because of imbalance—regardless of how active you are. This causes wear and tear on your joints, discs, ligaments, and other areas of your body. As you examine yourself in the mirror, I explain the proper alignment of your unique individual body.

Now that you have taken a general examination of your posture, you have the next seven chapters of section IV, Targeted Exercises, to refer to. These are the Bodysense therapy exercises for each part of the body. As a particular body problem gets aligned and strengthened, continue through the chapter and complete all the exercises.

The goal of this program is to be able to execute correctly the Level II exercises of the Total Fitness Daily Dozen Routine in section V. But the core of the book is in the Targeted Exercises, covering the body from toe to head. The exercises that are described as hazards and the potential problem exercises in the Personalized Total Fitness Test are discussed at length in the beginning of the chapter, and the corrective instruction for each are explained within the Targeted Exercises.

All the study and practice of the previous chapters lead into section V, the Bodysense Total Fitness Daily Dozen Routine. It consists of twelve exercises offering two levels of ability. Do not just flip to the back of the book and do what I call the Bodysense Daily Dozen. You will only be cheating yourself. Start from the beginning of the book, understand the Bodysense Method, be assured your body is aligned, and execute the exercise correctly. Then you can use the Total Fitness Daily Dozen Routine as a maintenance program.

I want you to be aligned not only while exercising, but also twenty-four hours a day. So section V also reviews Relaxation Techniques and Daily Living Habits such as sleeping, standing, sitting, driving, lifting, squatting, bending, leaning, push-pull, and shoveling. We often blame our jobs for giving us a pain in the back and neck, but it could well be the way we sleep at night or drive to work.

Just in case your excuse is you don't have the time to practice, I have set up five-, ten-, fifteen-, and thirty-minute programs.

Follow the program as I've outlined it for you. Pay strict attention to the details and the way you are executing the exercises.

Most students who are first exposed to the Bodysense Method come into the program with an accumulation of bad exercise habits. It's vital that you begin to break them and learn to practice the right approach. It's worth taking a little extra time and effort to study the Bodysense Method. If you make it a part of yourself, its positive effects will carry over into everything you do, and it will support your well-being for the rest of your life.

What are you *doing* to stay healthy? Notice I didn't ask what you know about good health. There is a big difference. I have always been puzzled that so many people take better care of their cars than they do of themselves. Remember, we become susceptible to diseases and injuries through neglect. A healthy body, balanced through the awareness of Bodysense, is more resistant to diseases and injuries.

So there's no excuse! Read on to learn about *Bodysense* and how to use it—for your body's sake.

3. Fundamentals

Our minds, bodies, and behaviors are all functionally inter-related, constantly influencing one another and interacting in a dynamic process. We are not made up of isolated, mechanical pieces. Our posture reflects our mood and, in turn, influences it. If you want to experience this, try walking around slump-shouldered for a few hours and see what happens to your mind and neck; they will reflect, reinforce, and intensify a stressful state. Eventually, the muscles will develop a stressful habit that can rob you of your natural vitality.

If, on the other hand, you knew how to maintain proper body alignment and increase your awareness of stress-related behavior, you could immediately begin to exercise greater control over your body and could alter it in a positive direction.

There are three types of habits that cause us to be misaligned:

1. Behavioral. These are our characteristic behaviors, such as working, eating, drinking, and social habits. They are the external patterns of behavior.
2. Physiological. These are our internal physiological patterns, such as breathing, circulatory, vascular, and other consistent patterns of activity in our internal environment.
3. Mental. These are the emotional/perceptual habits that are also the creative sources of stress.

The belief that we cannot, and do not, control certain parts of our bodies is false. The truth is that we have absolute control over our bodies. The problem lies in whether or not it is conscious or unconscious. Unconscious control means habit; conscious control means choice.

Developing physical consciousness is necessary to eliminate stress and can be a lot of fun. The key element is awareness; that is, removing the stress-producing habit patterns from the unconscious so that they can be altered. We suffer from prolonged stress primarily because of our habits, which are aggravated further by incorrect exercises. What allows these habits to continue to create and maintain constant stress is our lack of sensitivity to them and their consequences. Bodysense is an opportunity for us to stop our stressful habits and to exercise, walk, sit, stand, and participate in sports with balance and composure. You *can* learn to see, feel, understand, and eliminate the stressful habit patterns in your everyday life.

Here are the fundamentals of my technique:

- Rhythmic Breathing
- Alignment/Posture
- Stretching
- Concentration
- Discipline

Rhythmic Breathing

Few people breathe correctly, especially when they exercise. Many hold their breath, tense up, and strain. To function properly, all body cells must receive sufficient oxygen. The correct rhythmic breathing is: Inhale to get ready. Start to exhale and while contracting your abdominals, work into your exercise. Hold the position and continue breathing out five counts. Ease up on the exercise while inhaling. Then, exhale while working deeper into your exercise.

Executing deep rhythmic breathing is as basic to the Bodysense discipline as is the emphasis on special body alignment. It is the key that fabricates the mind and body together; the breath is the bridge between body and mind.

Deep breathing is nature's tranquilizer and rejuvenator. Providing sufficient oxygen to the system wards off fatigue and sluggishness. Slow, deep respiration reduces strain on the heart and blood vessels. Lungs well-exercised by proper breathing increase the body's ability to resist the common cold and other respiratory ailments.

The breath can be used as a tool to aid strength and endurance by promoting steadiness and harmony. Exhalation can be used to increase relaxation and stretch. Correctly contract your abdominals on exhalations to completely expel all of your breath. This is essential to a full inhalation. By directing the exhalation to areas of discomfort, the "stretch-not-strain pain" being experienced by body and mind during intense practice can be dissipated. Freedom from tension in the area being worked will allow the brain to be calm and the breath smooth.

Breathing is also influenced by one's mental state. When the mind is clear and balanced, the breath is even and rhythmic. When the mind is nervous and tense, the breath is strained and erratic. Watch for these things in your practice, and keep your breath flowing smoothly.

When learning a new pose and concentrating, one tends to hold the breath. Notice if you do this, and keep the breath moving. When holding the poses, breathe evenly, smoothly, and deeply. Inhaling increases strength and firmness in the muscles. Exhaling relaxes and softens them. Therefore, when twisting or stretching into a position, exhale slowly to make the muscles and the body pliable. This will prevent strain and allow you to go further into the exercise. I offer more breathing techniques in section III.

Alignment/Posture

Efficiency of motion is essential to good performance in sports. Each activity—walking, sprinting, long-distance running, jumping, and so forth—have specific, definable normal and abnormal motions. This is why an understanding of the particular sport's techniques and the mechanical abilities and limitations of the whole body's alignment are essential to a proper conditioning program.

Educating one's mind to the physical shortcomings of the body requires self-perception. It encompasses all aspects of activities: sleeping, walking, standing, eating, playing, and working.

People should not do athletics to get fit; instead, they should get fit and then do athletics. Of course, everybody wonders what that means. Let's take the average person who begins to exercise. If a person always walks with his feet out like Charlie Chaplin, he has a misalignment that probably stems from the hips or the knees. If someone walks with the feet out, he tends to run, stretch, and do strengthening exercises with the feet out. So the problem will only get worse as he exercises since he is reinforcing the misalignments.

You might never have given much thought to the importance of alignment. Yet, when a runner mentions the need of *balance,* she is really saying that her body needs to be *aligned* and that all the bones should line up in the way nature intended, rather than in the way we have come to let them because of our bad habits. When she mentions *flexibility* and *strength,* she is saying that the muscles surrounding those bones should be properly toned to control their alignment and allow for the optimum of freedom of motion. And, when she mentions *energy,* she is talking, in part, about the necessity of *breathing* correctly so the oxygen can get to all the working muscles and give them the stamina to run well and quickly.

Notice how the total picture as a runner sees it entails all the principles I'm speaking about in my explaination of the Bodysense Method.

Therefore, if you're misaligned (and who isn't), eventually you are going to run into trouble. Give yourself the Mirror Test in section III, chapter 2. When you play the guitar, you have to tune it first. Your body also needs tuning before playing sports. It may experience some discomfort as it gets properly conditioned, but do not get tense or resist—you will not break.

Stretching Technique

Sports Medicine is a relatively new science that shows there are *right* as well as *wrong* ways to go about the act of stretching one's body. Static stretching—the s-l-o-w, g-r-a-d-u-a-l pulling, holding, and releasing of specific muscle groups— has superseded ballistic-type calisthenics in the regimen of flexibility training for many athletes from grade school to the pros. Flexibility itself, for years the overlooked sibling of strength, endurance, and speed, has come to be appreciated for its own virtues. It is an aid to overall physical performance and a protection against muscle soreness and injury.

There are three important considerations that should be kept in mind during stretching. First, the stretch should be gentle and slow. If your movement is fast or forced, the muscle will react defensively to protect itself and tighten up. Hold your position for ten to sixty seconds to allow the muscle to adjust.

Second, don't lock your elbows or knees backward. This is called hyperextension and can lead to injury by interfering with the proper alignment and freedom in the stretch. So straight does not mean "locked."

To understand this, stand up, lean on one leg, and lock the knee backward. (Some people can do this more easily than others.) Notice that the leg feels shorter and that there is pressure in the back of the knee and very little awareness in the foot. This is what you should never feel again. Now, ease the knee to staighten the leg; raise the toes to press the ball of the foot into the floor; tighten the knee cap *upward*, not backward, to activate a lift and strength in the thigh muscle. If you have hyperextended knees, it is important that you apply this control at all times when stretching. The extension would be from the hip. For more information, read section IV, chapter 1.

The rule is the same for the arm. You should draw the elbow straight into alignment. To experience this, place your arm out to the side at shoulder level. Straighten the elbow, draw your shoulder blade downward, and squeeze inward, without resistance. Now, visualize someone pulling your fingertips. The focus of the stretch is from the shoulder girdle, and the extension is felt through the arm. See section IV, chapter 7 for more explanation.

Third, make sure you feel the stretch in the belly of the muscle. A lot of people stretch their legs without knowing where they should feel it. There are certain areas where you do not want to feel the stretch. They are at, or close to, the joints where there are mostly tendons and ligaments. Tendons are like rope, hardly able to stretch at all. If you pull on them, they will only become weakened. Ligaments hold bones together. When they are stretched, they cannot do their job. Loose and wobbly joints can cause many serious injuries.

Muscles can develop a particular type of chronic tension. A number of different conditions are responsible for this, including poor postural habits and emotional stress. When muscles are chronically tense, they become unnaturally hard and inflexible. They no longer have the suppleness to work effectively. Relaxation becomes difficult and energy is consumed at rest, even during sleep. The instinct would be to stretch these muscles; but their tightness severely reduces their capacity to stretch, and they will only tear or transfer the force to their tendons.

Stretching is also dangerous for torn muscles or tendons. They need rest and increased circulation to heal properly. A good method of increasing circulation and providing suppleness to a torn or tense muscle is a deep muscle massage. This done properly can help you regain and retain healthy muscles.

The difficult task is to give up the old stretching habits that might be ruining your future. For a time, it feels strange and even sacrilegious to alter your ritual; but new routines will become familiar and reward you with many more years of healthy activity.

Concentration

Most important, the method relies on concentration. To do the movements properly, you must pay attention to what you are doing. No part of your body is unimportant; no motion can be ignored.

Do not go into familiar exercises mechanically. I want you to be able to feel yourself in a sensory discovery of the way your body moves. I want you to understand that the movement of one part of your body is experienced by the entire body and that the body's unity comes from the simultaneous combination of movements, which do not contradict each other, but rather complement each other.

Forcing the body to act contrary to its unconscious reflexes accomplishes nothing—in any case, nothing of lasting value. As soon as your attention strays, the body resumes its old habits. What I try to do is make students aware of their structurally defective postures and actions that they have involuntarily executed for years. It's the sensory experience of the body that we're looking for, which can be accomplished by moving the intelligence and consciousness into all parts of the body.

Nothing should be stiff or jerky. Nothing should be too rapid or too slow. Smoothness and evenly flowing movement go hand in hand with control. Make sure you evaluate and correct any misalignments to execute the exercise properly. The minute you move out of alignment, you start pressing on blood, lymph, and nerve channels. This interferes with the efficiency and beauty of the body. When we move back into alignment, all those power lines loosen up.

Always stay on the threshold of your ability. Each body has its own threshold, which changes from day to day. Even an advanced student accumulates tightness and imbalances because modern life is governed by psychological stresses and physical inactivity: sitting, driving, and standing for long periods. Each day we must discover our thresholds, which are defined by the limits of flexibility and strength and are signaled by pain or immobility. As you approach your limit, your body will begin signaling you with mild pain. Don't force yourself through the pain. Stay just in back of it and move and breathe gently at your new threshold.

Discipline

Educating one's mind to the physical shortcomings of the body is an all-inclusive process. It encompasses all aspects of activities: sleeping, walking, standing, eating, lying, and working.

A budding pianist, when learning to play scales, does so awkwardly at first. Practice soon enables progression from scales to chords. Discipline, determination, and practice will influence the skill acquired. The same is true with Bodysense. Learning and practicing at a comfortable pace will enable the beginner to achieve modified basic poses and a gradual alignment of the body.

This method requires discipline. Combining internal concentration and breathing with the external flexing and contracting of the muscles can teach you to integrate the mind and body in a way that can benefit any activity that requires mental attention and physical ability.

Whether the goal of your training is to run for the pure pleasure of it or to be able to draw from your body that least bit of effort needed to win in competition, a basic knowledge of my techniques can aid and benefit you along the way.

Now, I would like to add a thought about relaxation. Relaxation has become nearly a lost art in our high-speed society. Physical tension affects the mind, just as a nervous, tense, or chattering mind affects the body. Each one reflects and becomes the other. Total relaxation cannot be achieved by simply resting or engaging in some diversion. Real relaxation—rejuvenation and renewal—is a positive state of balance and equilibrium in the body and mind and is attained through passive action. Real relaxation allows you to release pent-up energies, stored tensions, and energy blocks. It restores you to wholeness and makes it possible for you to experience well-being.

4. Procedures

Each exercise instruction is divided into the following categories:

- Props
- Body Placement
- Technique
- Variations
- Breathing Rhythm
- Tips
- Benefits

The instructions may seem long and complicated, but this is what distinguishes my book from other exercise books. I explain each exercise in detail and show visually the contrast or distinction between the correct and incorrect positions. This is a unique feature that enables the students to understand their own alignment, correct the misalignment, and then execute the exercise through the precise details. As you read the instructions and refer to the pictures, it is helpful to try to feel the action in your body and visualize the motion in your mind.

Props

The props used in this book are everyday household items (with the single exception of three-pound ankle weights), namely chairs, tables, doors, walls, and stairs. They are used in innovative ways to increase body strength and flexibility. The average person's home is already a mini-gymnasium; all he or she has to do is learn how to make use of it. Expensive equipment need not be purchased or rented to exercise correctly.

These props are only temporary aids to be used as a means of awakening and educating the body's natural intelligence. They are not crutches to be used for years on end. I suggest you alternate between using the prop and trying to work in exactly the same way without its aid.

Here is a list of the props. You can have them prepared, nearby, and ready to use.

1. Facecloth folded into eighths.
2. Facecloth folded in half and rolled up tight with rubber bands at each end to hold it together.
3. Magazine rolled up to measure an inch in diameter and held together firmly with rubber bands or a one-inch thick by twelve-inch long pole.
4. Two long neck ties tied together at the wide end and measuring approximately eight feet long.
5. 2½-foot long pole or the attachment from a vacuum.
6. Nylon belt with two rings to slide closed.

7. Small can (tunafish can in size) or a block of wood.
8. Unopened can of food that is 4½ inches high.
9. One set of three-pound ankle weights.
10. Full-length mirror for checking symmetry and alignment (important).

It is best to do the standing exercises on a hard, nonslip, level surface. The other exercises may be practiced on a blanket, mat, or carpet.

Body Placement

It is very important that you place your body correctly before you embark on the exercise. The placement is the foundation from which you work. Observe closely and follow the figure inserts provided. When standing, you must balance with a broad foot and lifted arches. To experience this, imagine you have four tires under your feet. Make sure they are aligned and balanced between the balls and heels.

When kneeling, the foundation is the center of the patella (kneecap). To make sure you are on the rim of the kneecaps, kneel with your knees hip-width apart. Then, without moving the knees on the floor, slide the kneecaps toward each other. This brings you to the rim of the kneecap with the ligament balanced. Read section IV, chapter 2 for more details of the Kneeling Thigh Tilt exercise.

When lying down on your back, balance between the two flat shoulder blades and level sacrum. To aid in attaining this balance, I suggest you lie down, bend your arms at the elbows, press the elbows into the floor, inhale, lift your chest, squeeze the shoulder blades together, then lower them. Take your hand and make sure your fingers can slide under your spine at the waist. This brings the spine into its natural lumbar curve and levels your sacrum. Read section IV, chapter 4 and section V, chapter 3 for more details.

When lying face down, balance between the two frontal hip-bones and pubic bone. Contract your abdominal muscles to attain this balance and firm foundation. Read section IV, chapter 5 for the Backward Flexion of the Back exercises.

When sitting, the proper placement is the solid foundation of the ischial (sit) bones. To find the correct angle, sit on a hard chair and slide to the edge until two bones roll off the edge of the chair. Back up the ischial bones so they are just one inch from the edge. Now, inhale, sit tall, and balance on the tips of your ischial bones. Notice the natural lumbar curve and the freedom in the lower back. The upper body has no strain. For more details, read sections IV and V, chapters 3.

Technique

The Technique portion is the core of the exercise, but do not skip past the Props and Body Placement for the Technique section. All parts of the Bodysense procedure are essential. The

Technique combines the breath and motion. It works the various body parts to expand your awareness, control, and body.

At first glance, all the instructions seem long and complicated. As you use them, however, you'll find that their precision plays a large part in the unique value of the Bodysense Method.

The photographs and figures are intended to help you understand the instructions quickly, completely, and accurately. When you are more experienced in the Method, they can be used as a quick reference and memory refresher. However, the photographs and figures do not give you enough information to do the exercises without reading the instructions.

Variations

Some people start out more limber or stronger than others. The Variations I offer are to satisfy people at many levels. Again, I want to emphasize that control and precision are more important than doing an exercise to the furthest point described in the Variations. You must never let go of your grounding technique in search of a more advanced goal. The main theme of the Bodysense Method is alignment and balance, and this should not be sacrificed. To simplify, I tell my students, "Analyze the position and keep in mind the part of the body that bears the weight on the floor has the priority of alignment. You then work up through the body without sacrificing your grounded base for the goal." When I say, "It's not how far you get that counts; it's how well you get there," I mean priority of purpose is alignment and balance.

Once more, I want to stress the importance of reading the instructions from the beginning and reviewing the Tips before executing the exercises

Breathing Rhythm

The Breathing Rhythm is the most important ingredient in the Bodysense Method. You will find the Breathing Rhythm routinely given in the Technique portion of the instructions. To clarify it further, it has been listed under its own heading. Never hold your breath while exercising—breathe freely. As a general rule, inhale to get ready, align the body, and perform the exercise on the exhale. Tension in breathing acts as a barometer in the exercising, revealing whether you are out of alignment or in an exercise that is too difficult for you. Pay attention to your breathing; it will keep you in touch with yourself.

Tips

The Tips are another important part of the instructions. They view the exercise as a whole and give specific beneficial pointers for just that exercise. Make sure you read the Tips portion before you begin the exercise. They are a result of my many years of experience. I know what people are apt to do wrong in these exercises, and the Tips can safeguard you from falling into the same pitfalls.

Benefits

The Benefits are listed to give you an overall idea what areas of the body the exercise is working. You will notice many Benefits as you practice. I found it hard to mention only a few, because each correctly executed exercise works on the whole body, inwardly and outwardly.

5. Miscellany

What to Wear

It is essential that you work with bare feet. Your shoes carry, reflect, and, therefore, reinforce all the imbalances of your body. Wearing socks can lead to slippage and inhibits observing the foot. Choose clothing that will not bind or restrict your movement or hinder you from viewing your knees, hips, and tummy. Do not wear baggy sweats or warm-up outfits; it is very difficult to find yourself.

For women, the best choice is a leotard with light-colored tights (Black makes it difficult to see the knees.) or a T-shirt and shorts.

For men, a T-shirt or tank top worn with comfortable shorts or swimming trunks is the best selection.

When to Exercise

Any time is a good time to exercise.

Regularity is the key to your Bodysense practice. Find some time that you will have available regularly in your day, perhaps a short session in the morning and a longer one in the evening. Morning sessions dissipate any sluggishness, improve mobility, and get the circulation going. They also make you alert so that the whole day goes better. Evening sessions relax and remove the tensions and imbalances accumulated during the day.

You should really practice six days out of seven; but, if that seems excessive, begin with every other day or four days a week. If this still seems demanding, try not to let a day go by without doing at least one of the corrective exercises you especially need to do.

Working with Injuries

Continue doing the Bodysense exercises that do *not* affect the injured area. Only when you have to use the injured part, review and apply the correct technique of alignment for that body area. Let's take for example, an injured ankle. You still have to walk with it, but placing weight on the foot at an angle inhibits the healing process. Balance the weight evenly by applying what I call the four tires. (See section IV, chapter 1.)

When you have an injury, get permission from a physician before stretching the injured area. Take this book to your doctor and show him or her what you intend to do.

In general, when you have an injury to muscles, ligaments, or tendons, do not stretch the area for three weeks, but keep it aligned. This gives it time to heal. Begin stretching the area by doing the easiest Bodysense exercise for that area. If the exercise causes pain, as opposed to a little stiffness, discontinue for another week. If it does not cause pain, practice this one exercise for two weeks. (It takes two to three weeks for an exercise to affect the body.) If the area continues to improve after this time, add another exercise. Do these two exercises for two weeks, then add a third, and so on. (If you add more than one exercise at a time, you will not know which exercise is good or bad for the injury.) Proper movement can be therapeutic if you work intelligently. Working this way may seem slow. Acknowledge your impatience, but know that methodical perseverance will pay off. If you are ambitious and push yourself too far too fast, you will have a constant reminder of your greed—continued pain.

Work at Your Own Level

I have designed this book for beginning, intermediate, and advanced students. The flow of exercises is planned so that each student can progress at his or her own pace. Keep in mind that it is not how far you advance in a given posture that is important, but that you perform each pose conscientiously. Gauge your progress solely against yourself, going only as far as you can while doing each exercise correctly. The Bodysense Method is noncompetitive. You are in total observation of yourself, as you gain feelings of freedom, rejuvenation, self-confidence, strength, and an innate sense that you are in control of your body; it does not control you.

Duration of Practice

Set aside some time during the day when you can practice undisturbed. Fifteen to twenty minutes a day is usually adequate in the beginning. An experienced student should spend at least an hour a day on his or her practice. This includes breathing exercises and relaxation.

While practicing, the position should be held for ten to fifteen seconds in the beginning. As your body gains flexibility and strength, slowly begin to increase the length of holds. Generally, the position should be held from thirty seconds to one minute. Gradually increase the period and/or repeat the exercise from the beginning. Don't hold a position beyond your ability to come out of it with control.

How Many Repetitions

Mechanical, robot-like action will not be possible if you are attentive in your practice. The exercises are done a few times each, usually only three to five times. But what's different is you hold the position for awhile. As you direct the integration of breathing and movement, you will develop a sense of rhythmical balance. Once you have learned the basic rhythm, you can begin the real exploration with emphasis on *doing* and *being*. This exciting discovery of self bypasses the boring aspect of other mechanically repetitious routines.

Good Practice Habits

- As I said in the previous section, always practice attentively. Don't do the exercises half-consciously or mechanically. Be attentive to the position of all bodily parts: the correct movements, breathing, alignment, and symmetry.

- Go as far into the stretch as you can while maintaining the alignment described. It is more beneficial to do the pose with correct alignment than to sacrifice the structure so that you *appear* to be stretching further. You should be on the "edge" of your stretch, that is, "very aware" of the muscles you are working; without being in pain. Pain has a stringy sensation; but being "very aware" feels like a wide, long, warm area. If you are lazy, changes will not occur; if you are overly ambitious, you will get hurt.

- Never exercise unprepared or "cold" muscles; you might tear tissues or muscles. You will get better performance with minimum effort after you do the basic warm-ups your individual body needs to bring it into alignment. Your body will feel warm and loose, ready for specific, concentrated postures.

- Do not bounce. The conglomerate of exercise program offered these days tends to focus on achieving a goal, such as touching the toes ten times. The Bodysense Method places much less emphasis on goals. Rather, it encourages students to finely tune the manner in which they move. The extreme concentration and close observation requires drawing the attention inward, which quiets and integrates the mind and body.

- Do the exercises with a slow, smooth, and coordinated approach. Movements should flow with rhythmically controlled breathing. Although some of the postures may appear passive or relaxed, they are actually positive and dynamic. Slowly stretching muscles to full length and then holding them in absolute stillness causes blood to circulate evenly throughout the body. This brings every muscle group into plan and allows the range of movement to be increased in all muscles, ligaments, tendons, and joints. Bodysense especially increases spinal flexibility by stretching.

- You must never strain to attain a position in which your body is uncomfortable. If you do so, you will actually retard your progress. While practicing, you must listen to your body. It will tell you what condition it is in. If you start off by doing too much, you will only fatigue the body. Ideally, a workout of ten to fifteen minutes every day is far better than one hour once a week. Many people, when feeling limited in a particular area, tighten up the surrounding muscles in an attempt to protect the tight area. They are tensing and straining the area rather than relaxing and opening it through proper control and balance.

- Some soreness is normal when the muscles are being toned and strengthened to new limits and when new sets of muscles are being used. Do not favor that area and throw your posture out of line—maintain your alignment. Relief can be had by a hot bath, mild stretching, or a good, deep massage. The best treatment, however, is regular practice.

- You will probably notice that one side of your body does not respond as quickly as the other. You have what we call a "good" side and a "bad" side. Sometimes it is helpful to do the bad side twice. We also tend to avoid certain exercises, and these are most likely the ones we need to do the most. Don't you want to gain a well-balanced, conditioned body?

- As you progress in ability and understanding, reread the detailed instructions from time to time. Once you have gained experience, you will have a different perspective and be better able to absorb details. Above all, enjoy your new found Self.

Section II

Two Important Tests

1. *Hazards*
2. *Personalized Total Fitness*

To test your Bodysense, check off the exercises you think are correct!

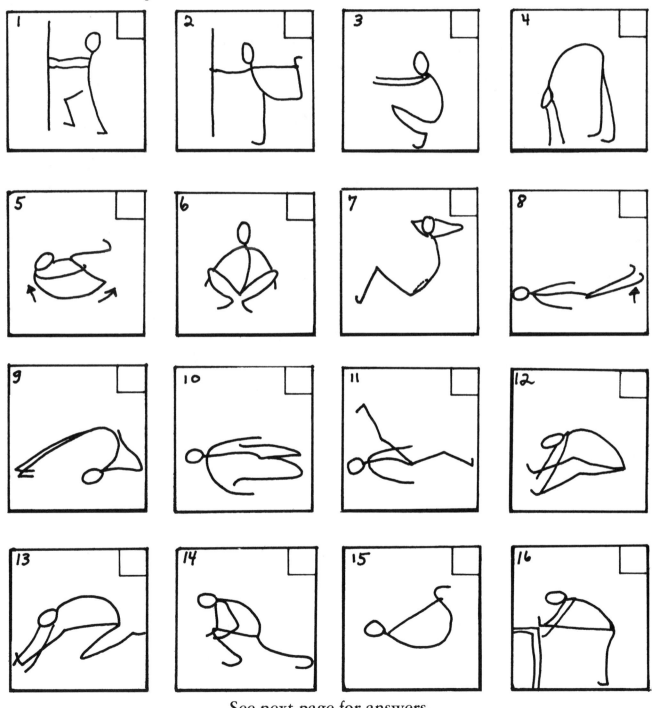

See next page for answers.

1. Hazards

THEY ARE *ALL* HAZARDOUS WAYS OF EXERCISING!

These traditional exercises are practiced fervently by conscientious people. Since they have been around for awhile, it is assumed that they must be worthwhile, even if they often feel uncomfortable and provide little or no sign of increased flexibility. With the lack of detailed instructions, breathing techniques, and warnings, the individual with the no-pain-no-gain attitude plunges into the position and assumes if it hurts it must be doing good.

I see this daily. Athletes, weekend jocks, and regular exercise buffs work diligently at their exercises, paying attention to one part of the body to the detriment of the rest and knowing nothing of their personal alignment patterns and body limitations. They are reinforcing their misalignment and doing more harm than good to their bodies. They are stretching, but stretching incorrectly.

So their problem worsens as they do warm-up exercises. The continued aggravation causes them harm and eventually hampers them from enjoying the sport itself. Unfortunately, one tries to achieve an instant goal without being aware of the body's needs along the way. This book has been written to cultivate your *Bodysense*.

BODYSENSE CORRECTIONS

1. Achilles, Ankle, and Calf Stretch

This stretch is meant to work the areas the name implies, but the lower back gets the strain even before the lower leg receives the action. Most students lean into the stretch, thinking that is it. Wrong! They are rolling their ankle to either side and putting strain in the ankle joint. The foot is twisted, and most likely the knee is turned or hyperextended. See section IV, chapter 1 for more detail on the balanced foot position.

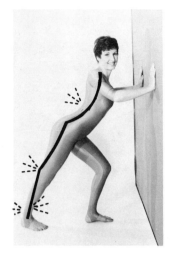 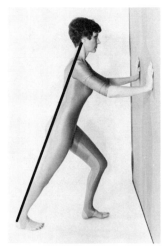

INCORRECT   **CORRECT**

2. Quadricep Stretch

It is meant to work the front of the thighs. The lower back, hip, and knees are really aggravated before the thighs get their stretch, and the back is compressed. See section IV, chapter 2.

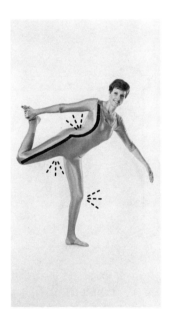 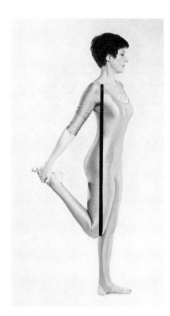

INCORRECT   **CORRECT**

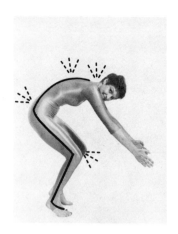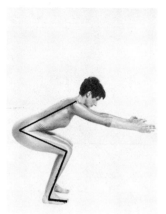

3. Deep Knee Bend

This exercise is the cause of many knee injuries. It puts enormous pressure on the cartilage in the knee because the knees have very poor footing; that is, the ankles roll in or out, and the feet are not grounded to support the knee. In addition, the back is rounded and bent forward. See section IV, chapter 1.

INCORRECT   **CORRECT**

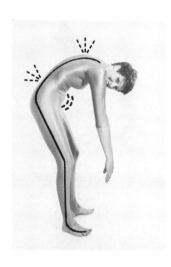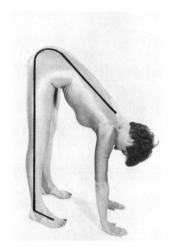

4. Toe-Touching Stretch

This puts enormous strain on the lower back. When bending with a rounded back, your back muscles are not supported; you are actually hanging by your ligaments. The abdominal muscles are not contributing to the support of the hips. This puts great stress on the spine, sciatic nerve, and discs. The back pain often does not set in until hours later, so the connection with this stretch is not noticed. This is a very common and serious problem stretch. See section IV, chapter 5.

INCORRECT   **CORRECT**

5. Back and Hip Stretch

This is another exercise given as a back "relaxer." For those whose spines do not roll on the floor, this might give temporary relief. But for most, the muscles are pulling away from the spine, making the spine protrude backward. This adds a great deal of stress to the ligaments and muscles of the back, sciatic nerve, discs, and neck. See section IV, chapter 2.

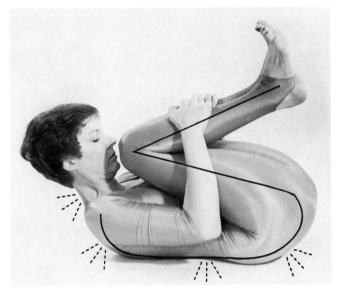

INCORRECT

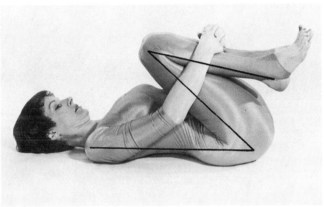

CORRECT

6. Groin Stretch

If you are sitting with your knees way up in the air and back rounded, you are not reaching your groin but aggravating your hips and lower back and putting a lot of pressure into the knees. Never "push" your knees to the floor while doing this stretch. Read section IV, chapters 2 and 3.

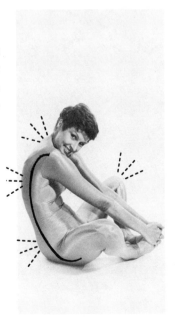

INCORRECT

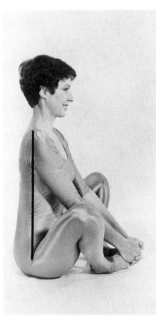

CORRECT

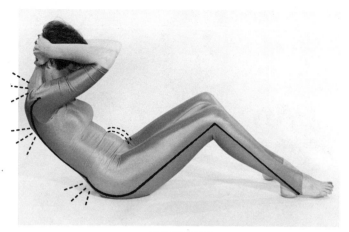

INCORRECT

7. Sit-Ups

Doing Sit-Ups with momentum will result in back strain—if not when you're young, then in later years. Put your hand on your abdomen. If it protrudes, you are straining your back and actually creating a protruded hard abdomen (even if your knees are bent). Sit-Ups are a very common cause of back and groin pain and the inability to acquire a flat abdomen. Read section IV, chapter 4.

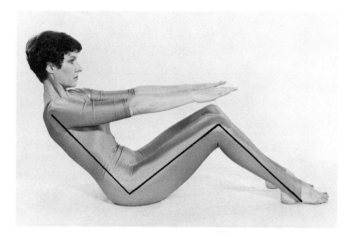

CORRECT

8. Double-Stiff Leg Raise

Even done correctly, this exercise puts a tremendous strain on the lower back. The abdominals are definitely straining outward. I do not teach this exercise, nor do I recommend that it be practiced. See section IV, chapter 4 for instructions on how to work the abdominals correctly.

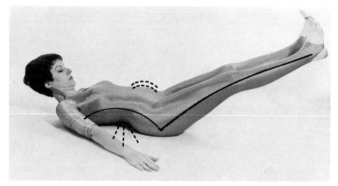

INCORRECT

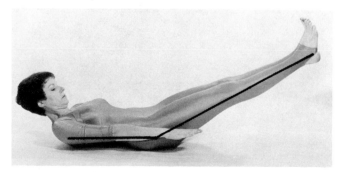

CORRECT

9. Plow

When the plow is performed with a round back it is very destructive to the neck. The plow compresses the blood vessels to the brain, upper spinal cord, and chest. It strains the whole length of the spine, literally tearing the ligaments in the back and adding injury to the sciatic nerve. The plow might feel good when you do it; but with continued incorrect practice, you are sowing the seed for serious problems. Read section IV, chapter 3 to learn how to use your body correctly without putting such strain on the neck or back.

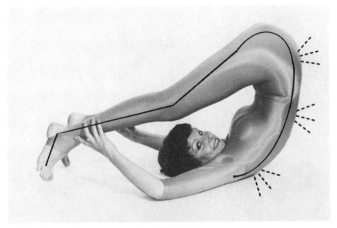

INCORRECT

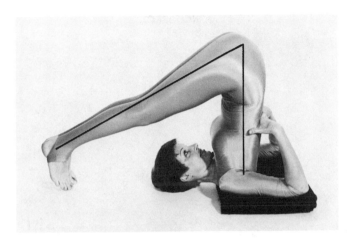

CORRECT

10. Thigh Stretch

It should be called knee stretch, because it strains the ligaments of the knees before the thighs get the action. When you lower to the floor without first rotating the pubic bone upward, the lower back is pinched. This causes strain or jam. Review section IV, chapters 2 and 5.

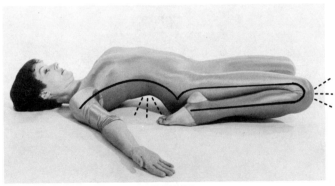

INCORRECT

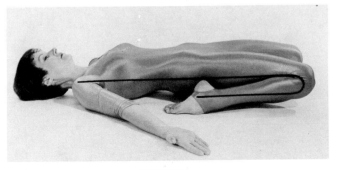

CORRECT

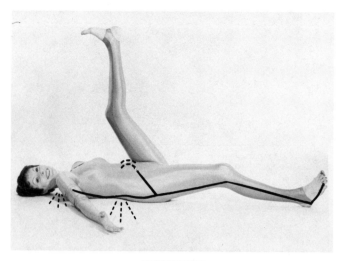

INCORRECT

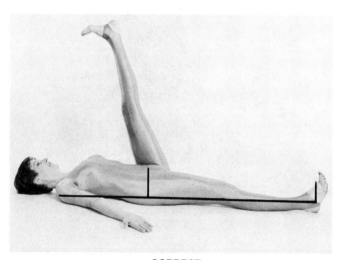

CORRECT

11. Single-Leg Raise

This stretch is rarely done with a straight leg. Most often it is done by pressing the spine into the floor with the knee bent, which puts a strain in the lower back, hips, and neck. When lifting the leg up, a tremendous drag and pull is added to the back and hips. Read section IV, chapters 2 and 3.

12. Sitting Forward Bend

This exercise is supposedly performed for stretching the hamstrings; but before the hamstrings even get a stretch, the back is greatly aggravated by the rounded-back posture. When you pull yourself forward with a rounded back and the hips jammed backward, you're literally tearing back ligaments and possibly creating injury to the sciatic nerve. See section IV, chapter 3.

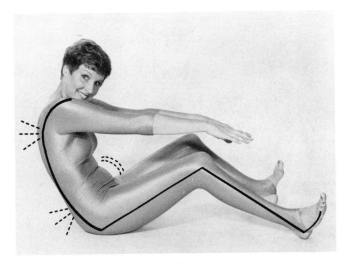

INCORRECT

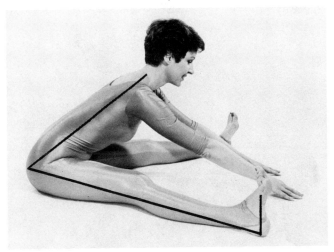

CORRECT

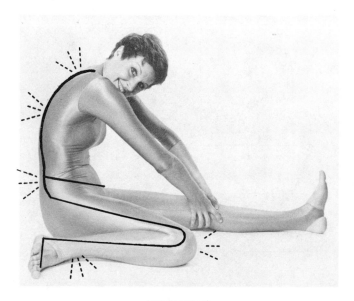

INCORRECT

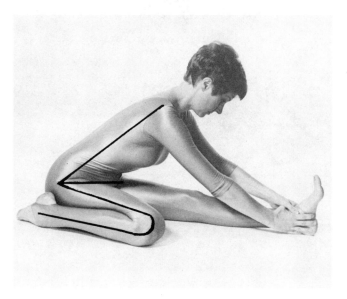

CORRECT

13. Hurdler's Stretch

When performed with a rounded back and the hips locked backward and unevenly (not sitting evenly on the floor), this exercise stretches the groin region farther than it is normally intended to go. This creates groin pulls. What I find sad is you think your groin is too tight, so you continue to practice the Hurdler's Stretch and aggravate it even more. This exercise also puts tremendous unnatural pressure sideways against the inner ligaments of the bent knee, adding stress and endangering the stability in the knee joint. It is also bad for the hips and lower back. See section IV, chapters 2 and 3.

14. Lunge Groin Stretch

When you lunge the knee beyond the ankle and the foot is not grounded, you add a lot of tension and strain in the knee, joints, and ligaments. In addition, a tremendous drag on the hips is created, because they are always uneven. Yes, you do get a stretch in the groin, but you are also hanging in the hip, twisting in the groin, and pinching in the lower back. See section IV, chapters 2 and 5 to learn how to stretch the groin correctly.

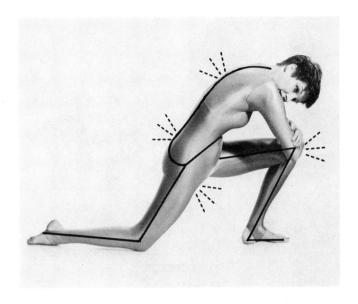

INCORRECT

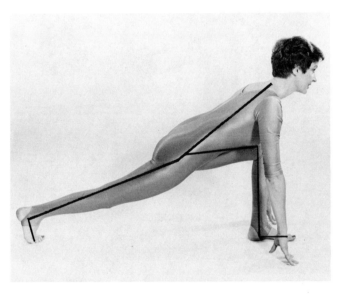

CORRECT

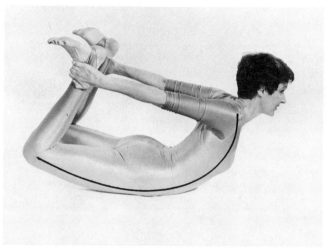

INCORRECT

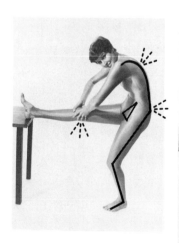

INCORRECT

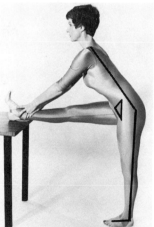

INCORRECT **CORRECT**

15. Bow Backarching

In this exercise and other backarching exercises, you work only at bending the back backward, which puts a tremendous amount of pressure on the lumbar discs four and five; it literally folds them together. This also puts a lot of tension in the neck and shoulder joints. Later in the day, you wonder why your back aches and pain is going down your leg. For the answer, read section IV, chapter 5 on the Backward Flexion of the Back.

16. Leg-Up Stretch

This is a very advanced stretch; but everyone does it, hoping someday he or she will succeed. It is doing you more damage than good. Hanging in the leg with the knee unsupported jams the knee backward, which causes posterior knee injuries to those with hyperextended knees. The exercise is done to stretch the hamstrings; but, instead, you're liable to tear it. If your leg is too high, you are injuring the hip joint as well. Again, this rounded-back posture is straining the lumbar ligaments and failing to actually stretch the hamstrings. Read section IV, chapter 2.

2. *Personalized Total Fitness*

If you have found it difficult to execute the correct versions of these exercises, take the Personalized Total Fitness Test to discover the areas on which you need to work.

This evaluation sheet will show you, at a glance, the areas that need work. Go to the appropriate chapter for further training, align and strengthen your weak areas, then repeat the test and check your improvement. Work with the chapter and corresponding chapter areas until you pass the test. Good luck!

Ten Tests	Needs Work	Accomplished
1. Balancing on Balls of Feet See section IV, chapter 1		
2. Balancing on One Leg See section IV, chapter 1		
3. Squatting Balance See section IV, chapter 1		
4. Standing Forward Bend See section IV, chapter 5		
5. Sit Balance See section IV, chapter 3		
6. Sitting Forward Bend See section IV, chapter 3		
7. Backward Arching See section IV, chapter 5		
8. Sit-Up See section IV, chapter 4		
9. Squeeze Spine into Body See section IV, chapter 2		
10. Leg Raise See section IV, chapters 2 & 3		

BODYSENSE CORRECTiONS

1. Balancing on Balls of Feet

Benefits	Working the feet into alignment with the body is the most important factor in acquiring good posture.
Directions	Balance up on the balls of the feet and keep the feet parallel. Hold for ten seconds. You should feel pressure on the ball of the big toe to the little toe.
Incorrect Movements	Are you rolling to the outside of the feet?
Potential Problems	A general lack of body alignment is indicated when the feet must "lock" outward to ensure balance. The ankles are strained, knees are locked backward, belly is thrust out, and buttocks is back—watch out!

Needs Work—See section IV, chapter 1.

Accomplished—Good for you!

2. Balancing on One Leg

Benefits	Balance is achieved through alignment, not compensation. The body is in its aligned position and not merely struggling to stay upright by contortions.
Directions	Stand straight on one leg without holding onto something. Hold still for ten seconds. Remember to feel for equal pressure across the ball of the foot and keep the pressure equal also between the ball and heel (balance).
Incorrect Movements	Are you wiggling all over and looking for something to hold on to?
Potential Problems	Alignment is sacrificed in an attempt to lower the center of gravity and achieve balance. The body literally collapses about itself. The knees are bending, hips are moving to the side, arms are extended, and back is rounded—watch out!

Needs Work—See section IV, chapter 1.

Accomplished—Well done!

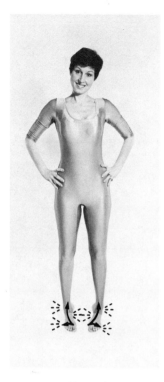

Figure 1

Figure 2

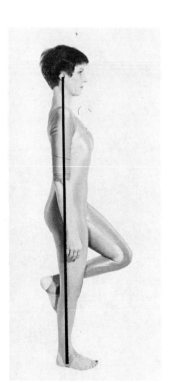

Figure 1

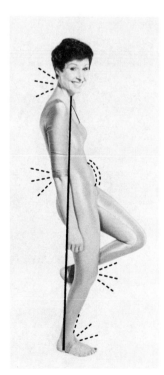

Figure 2

3. Squatting Balance

Benefits

The low back, calf muscles, and thighs are being both stretched and strengthened in a posture that also demands balance.

Directions

Can you squat down with a straight back, balancing on the balls of your feet, as in figure 1? With a slight tilt, lower onto your heels, as in figure 2. Hold for five seconds and come up as slowly as you came down. Remember to balance and align your feet, and keep your back straight and relaxed.

Incorrect Movements

Are your feet waddling and your body leaning forward, as in figure 3? When it is time to lower onto your heels, do you find yourself lifting up your buttocks, as in figure 4? Or have you fallen over, as in figure 5?

Potential Problems

Excessive pressures are being transferred to the knees and ankles. There is no coordination between the lower back, leg strength, and movement. There is a loss of balance and alignment, the knees are jammed, the back is rounded, and your weight is uneven on your feet—watch out!

Needs Work—See section IV, chapter 1.

Accomplished—Bravo!

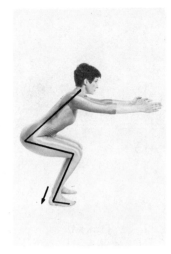
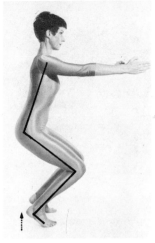

Figure 1

Figure 2

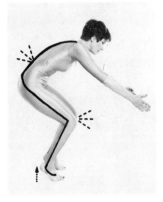
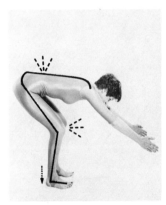

Figure 3

Figure 4

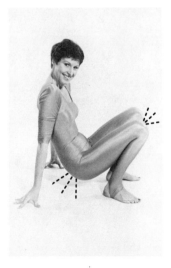

Figure 5

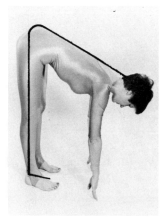

Figure 1

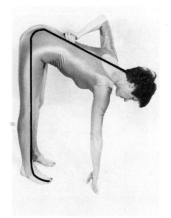

Figure 2

4. Standing Forward Bend

Benefits	The raised buttocks removes "slack" from the hamstrings and prepares the muscles for a well-controlled stretch. The head and chest slightly raised places the lower back in a strong strain-free alignment.
Directions	Can you bend forward, keeping your legs and back straight, as in figure 1? Check with your fingers, as in figure 2, to see if your spine is nestled into a slight groove down the center of your back. "Extend" (elongate) your spine, bend forward as you exhale, and remember to rotate your buttocks upward and stretch the hamstrings behind your thighs.
Incorrect Movements	Is figure 3 the only way you can bend over? Feel the spine rounding out of your back. Do your knees hyperextend, as in figure 4? In order to touch the floor, do you have to bend your knees, as in figure 5?

**Potential
Problems**

By bending in this manner, the muscles of the lower back are being stretched well beyond their optimum point. Worse, they are required to support the entire weight of the upper body like a counter lever. Eventually, this could lead to a significant weakening of the lower back. Hyperextension of the knee is traumatic to the synovial capsule and to the ligaments of the joint. In addition, all standing postures require that strength and control come from the body stance. "Locked legs" prohibit this and tension is greatly increased on the neck, shoulders, and back. This is the most common error and greatly increases back problems—watch out!

Needs Work—See section IV, chapter 5.

Accomplished—Well done!

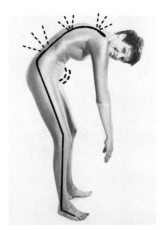

Figure 3

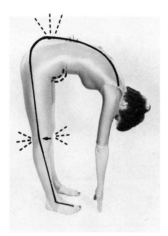

Figure 4

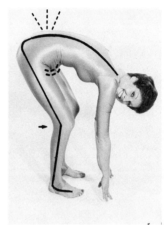

Figure 5

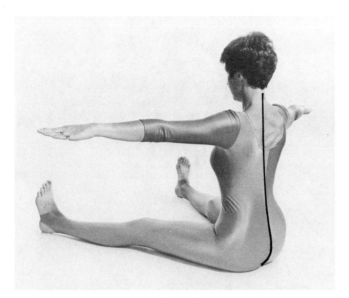

Figure 1

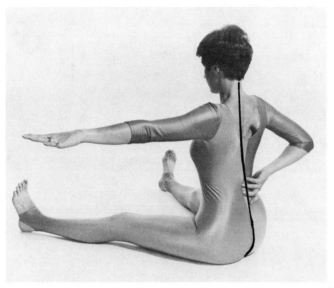

Figure 2

5. Sit Balance

Benefits   The low back and abdominal muscles work together to support the upper body in a two-column position—the spine behind and the abdominal muscles in front. The hamstrings are efficiently stretched, and the entire body is balanced.

Directions   Can you sit up with a straight back, with your legs stretched out front, as in figure 1? Feel your back to check if you have maintained a smooth groove, as in figure 2. The muscles are supporting your spine correctly only if you don't feel the bones of your spine sticking out.

Incorrect Movements	Do you find yourself with a bowed back, as in figure 3? Check for that spine sticking out! When you work the spine into the body and straighten the back, do your legs have to bend, as in figure 4?
Potential Problems	Inability to perform this posture correctly is the surest indication of tight hamstrings. Allowing the back to collapse only compresses the chest and ruins well-controlled breathing. Forcing a forward bend with a rounded back, then straining the lumbar ligaments and muscles causes back pain—watch out!

Needs Work—See section IV, chapter 3.

Accomplished—Good for you!

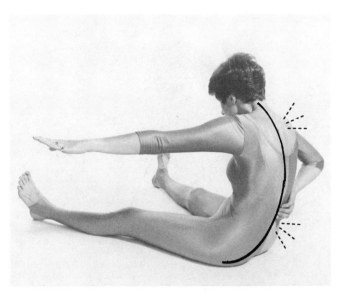

Figure 3

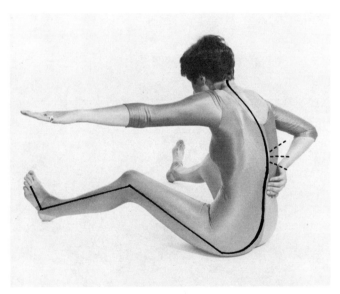

Figure 4

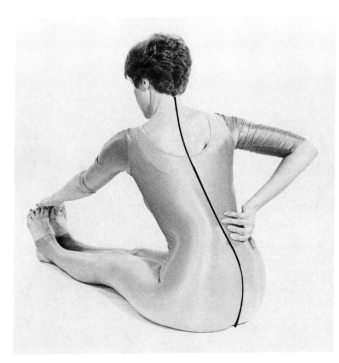

Figure 1

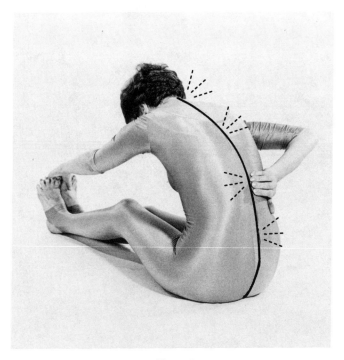

Figure 2

6. Sitting Forward Bend

Benefits

As you bend forward from the Sit Balance position, the chest and throat are open, the spine is extended (elongated), and the abdomen is supported rather than compressed by the upper body. Free, comfortable but controlled, breathing is the foundation of all postures.

Directions

Can you bend forward from the hips, maintaining a straight back without bending your legs? Hold for five seconds while holding onto the toes. Check to see if the spine is aligned and not popping out.

Incorrect Movements

Do you find yourself bending your legs to touch your toes? Feel that back again to see how you are bending. Is the stretch coming from forcing the back outward (rounded)?

Potential Problems

This position manages only to take the slack out of the body. No real stretch is taking place. If you continue to bounce or pull in this manner, you may create a weak and vulnerable back. You can overstretch the lumbar ligaments and muscles. This collapses the chest and abdomen—watch out!

Needs Work—See section IV, chapter 3.

Accomplished—Good control!

7. Backward Arching

Benefits   Working the abdominals correctly *elongates* the spine and prevents pinching in the lower back.

Directions   With your face down, can you arch the ribs and legs off the floor without feeling strain in the lower back? Extend and elongate the spine.

Incorrect Movements   Is it difficult for you to get your ribs and thighs off the floor, as in figure 2? Or are you raising only one end up at a time, as in figures 3 and 4? Do you feel pinching in the lower back?

Potential Problems   Inability to perform this posture implies weakness in the spinal muscles, buttocks, and abdominals. The danger in forcing it incorrectly is in compressing the spine and straining the muscles—watch out!

Needs Work—See section IV, chapter 5.

Accomplished—Bravo!

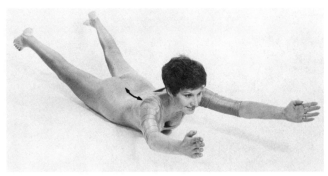

Figure 1

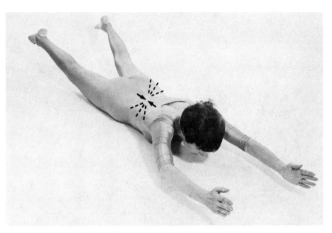

Figure 2

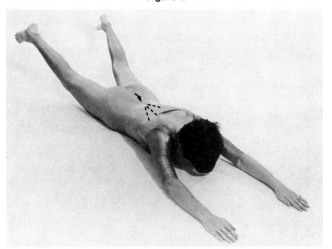

Figure 3

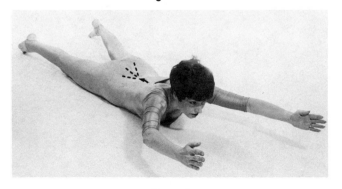

Figure 4

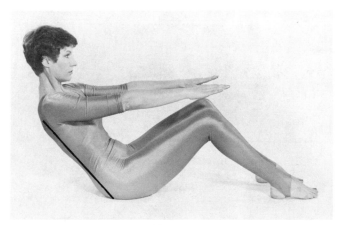

Figure 1

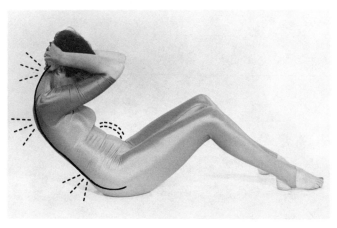

Figure 2

8. Sit-Up

Benefits

"Power moves" require special attention of form. With the abdominal wall intact, raising and lowering slowly can be performed with smooth control, and a strong, *flat* abdomen will be developed. This is critical for a strong back.

Directions

Can you slowly roll up and down from the floor without your abdominal muscles popping forward (bulging)? Breathe in, begin the Sit-Up as you exhale, while contracting the front abdominal muscles inward and upward. Keep elongating your spine and keep it straight as you come up.

Incorrect Movements

Do you thrust your body up while leading with a hard, protruded abdomen? Do you have to anchor your feet under a support to get up?

Potential Problems

When only a portion of the abdominal muscles are used to perform a Sit-Up, the result will be a protruded abdomen. The work is actually being accomplished by the deep back muscles called the psoas, which will become tight and cause hip and lower back tightness and malalignments—watch out!

Needs Work—See section IV, chapter 4.

Accomplished—Very good!

9. Squeeze Spine into Body

Benefits Done correctly, this elongation of the spine does more than move the hips; it *works* the hips with full flexion.

Directions Can you arch the spine off the floor as you use your knee for leverage? Keep the sacrum and shoulder blades flat on the floor. The leg on the floor must remain straight to elongate the spine

Incorrect Movements Do you recognize yourself, as in figure 2?—with a rounded spine pressing into the floor, the other leg wanting to bend at the knee, and the buttocks rolling up off the floor?

Potential Problems With the bending of the knee, the pelvis is no longer anchored. No true stretch of the hip is possible, because the pelvis rotates and rolls upward as you try to pull your thigh onto your chest—watch out!

Needs Work—See section IV, chapter 2.

Accomplished—Good work!

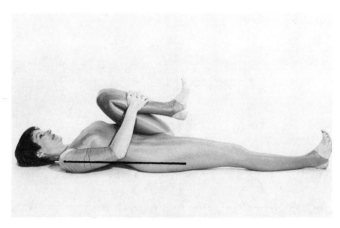

Figure 1

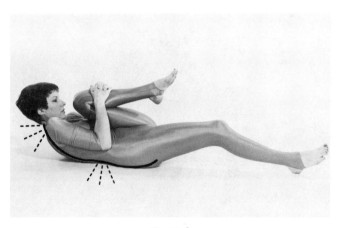

Figure 2

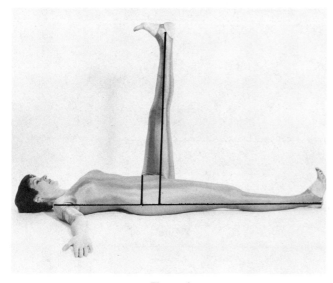

Figure 1

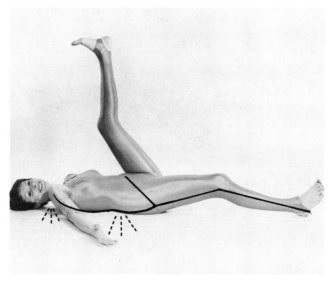

Figure 2

10. Leg Raise

Benefits	Proper form results in an efficient stretch of the hamstrings and calf muscles. The neck is free of stress, shoulders are flat, and the pelvis is well anchored.
Directions	Can you raise your leg straight up without bending either leg? Your spine should not be pressing into the floor. Hold for five seconds.
Incorrect Movements	Do you find yourself, as in figure 2 rounding your back and pressing the spine into the floor. You are straining your neck, and your tight hamstrings are preventing you from straigtening your legs.
Potential Problems	The bent knee and tilted pelvis compromise the stretch. Extreme tension is placed on the neck muscles. Their mechanical disadvantage is similar to trying to hold a bowling ball at arms length—watch out!

Needs Work—See section IV, chapters 2 and 3.

Accomplished—Good sport!

Section III

Fundamentals of Bodysense

1. *Proper Breathing Techniques*
2. *Proper Body Alignment*

1. Proper Breathing Techniques

"And the Lord, God, formed man of the dust of the ground and breathed into his nostrils the breath of life, and man became a living soul." (Genesis 2:7) All life is breath, and without breath there is no life.

Yoga is the source of my study of breathing. Deep, rhythmic breathing is the first lesson in Yoga and is basic to all its teaching. Breathing feeds the body's tissues, organs, and glands with oxygen; removes much of body waste; and maintains good health, aiding in resistance to disease and glandular balance. Deep breathing has a beneficial influence on the mind and emotions by relaxing the mind, clearing the memory, and promoting mental stability. In addition to these physiological and psychological benefits, breath control helps us gain a certain degree of mastery over our minds and bodies; for with each deep breath, we incorporate a burst of energy, which expands our self-expression and confidence as well as the lungs.

The breath is the external manifestation of the life force. It is our very life. We can live for awhile without food or drink, but not without the breath.

Learning how to breathe properly is basic to the performance in sports, gymnastics, dancing, and all exercise programs; but, unfortunately, proper breathing is often neglected in physical training curricula. The nonathletic person also needs proper breathing. The educated inhalation nourishes starved tissue and helps to normalize weight in those who are overweight or underweight; the proper exhalation aids the body in ridding itself of wastes that have accumulated as fat or toxins.

Breathing is really a very complex activity that can have a direct effect on many bodily functions. The pattern of our breathing—whether we breathe rapidly or slowly, deeply or shallowly, or whether we breathe through only the left or right nostril—could well determine our susceptibility to illness, the strength of our hearts, and the depths of our depressions.

Breathing is the way in which we transport oxygen from the air to our bodies' cells, where it is used to burn carbohydrates, proteins, and fats. This releases the energy that keeps us going. It is also the way in which we rid our bodies of a byproduct of the combustion process, carbon dioxide.

In a normal breath, we take in and give out about one pint of air. If we use a little force, by inhaling and exhaling deeply, we can take in and expel another three pints of air. The lung capacity is ten pints. So, you can imagine the amount of extra oxygen and life force you can get by deep breathing.

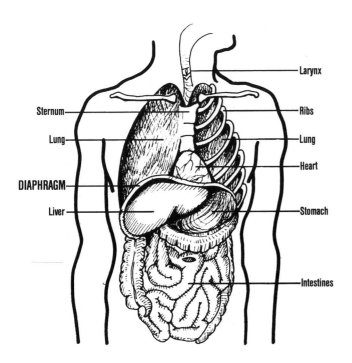

Sternum

Lung

DIAPHRAGM

Liver

Larynx

Ribs

Lung

Heart

Stomach

Intestines

We take breathing so much for granted that we often fail to recognize how inadequately and inefficiently we breathe. Breathing is one of the few body functions that usually operates at an unconscious level, but that can be brought under direct conscious control.

Emotional states influence breathing patterns markedly. Breathing reflects inner emotions: we gasp in amazement and pain, choke with sadness, hold our breath in anticipation, and sigh with relief. We feel breathless with excitement or inspired by an idea. Our breathing halts in fear or becomes irregular and ragged with anger. One way to inhibit feelings is by restricting breathing, and one way to release feelings is by freeing breathing. In each case, the way we feel—physically and emotionally— is directly linked to the way we breathe. Breathing has always been taken for granted by Western science.

Little has been said or written about the energy and endurance produced by breathing *correctly*. Much has appeared on how running or swimming eventually improves physical endurance; but the real key to physical power is not how many miles you run in a day, but how well you breathe. Learn to breathe fully and endurance is yours, whenever you want it.

Everyone breathes, but how? We can best understand how to breathe correctly by assessing the implications and results of shallow or improper breathing.

To start with, let's first dispel a common misconception on breathing. Do not breathe by blowing out or distending what you think of as your stomach. Actually, the stomach is located below the ribs, slightly left of center. There are no lungs below the rib margin, so why create pressure by forcing the breath downward when you can relax the abdomen and let the diaphragm do its job? The diaphragm works like a bellows. It is attached to the rib cage and is a flat muscle leaf, which separates the lungs from the abdomen.

The stomach is *not* down in the belly or tummy, as it is often thought to be; our intestines are housed there. If you place the palm of your hand in that sensitive opening between the ribs, you will feel the action of the diaphragm going up and down. Remember, do *not* inflate your tummy, belly, or abdominals when breathing. They should remain relaxed on inhale and contract inward on exhale to aid the diaphragm's expulsion of air upward and out.

Most people breathe either by sniffing their nose or keeping their mouths open. Both kinds of breathing are very shallow and lead to oxygen starvation of various parts of the body. They never get a deep, full breath; at best it is a casual breath.

I've long thought that the relaxation derived from smoking was not from the nicotine but rather from the deep breathing that smokers use to inhale cigarette smoke. Better for us all if we learn how to take an oxygen drag without the nicotine and toxic smoke.

I'd like you to take an honest, good, deep breath. What was your first reaction—was it to sniff, or did you open your mouth? Really concentrate and actively follow along with this chapter.

It will be the most important thing you can do for yourself.

When breathing correctly, you force the air to pass through your nose. There is no sensation in the nose; it stays relaxed and open and functions as a filtering passageway or tunnel. As you are reading this, concentrate on keeping the nose relaxed, and draw your attention to the inside of your mouth.

The two spots of consciousness for good breathing are the *larynx* in the hollow center of the collarbone and the *diaphragm* at the base of the ribs.

The diaphragm is a broad, flat, dome-shaped muscle that separates the thoracic (chest) cavity from the abdominal cavity. It is our principle breathing muscle and can be used and trained as other muscles. Unfortunately, in the majority of people, tension in and around the abdominal region and bad posture restrict diaphragmatic breathing so much that the resulting capacity to breathe is possibly one-third to one-quarter of what it could be.

I've made you aware of the opening in your throat, in which the breath passes through, and the diaphragm muscle, which draws the air in and pumps it out. Now, we will go through an exercise where the two work together.

Imagine your breath to be like an elevator, the diaphragm being its generator. It works downward like a suction pump, creating a vacuum that draws the breath from the nose through the larynx. Remember, the nose does not bring in the breath, it is a filtering passageway only. As the air is drawn in, the lungs start to inflate, like two balloons. The mid-rib area acts like an accordion, expanding outward on the inhale. You cannot force the accordion open or shut, so do not rush your inhale. Finally, air reaches the upper lobes of the lungs. Here, you should not force the ribs up (out), rather you should concentrate on the sternum. Place your finger on the center of the sternum. Stretch the skin upward and feel the chest really open up. Your shoulders should go backward instead of tensing toward your ears. Pause your breath at the end of inhalation, before you exhale.

Like inhalation, the diaphragm generates exhalation. During exhalation, the breath is expelled by the upward motion of the diaphragm. The recoil of the rib cage forces the air to escape through the upper airways. At this time, the shoulders roll back and downward, and the lungs (balloons) deflate, as the rib cage compresses around them (the action of the accordion).

To facilitate expelling all the stale air out of the body, contract your abdominal muscles inward and upward. This will also aid the diaphragm in its job. Pause briefly before beginning the next inhale cycle.

I don't call my breathing diaphragmatic because diaphragmatic breathing, as it is commonly taught, is the pushing out of the intestines (letting your belly blow up). I call my technique the Complete Breath or Rib Cage Breathing.

"Our life should be measured by breath rather than years," say David Stuart Sobel and Faith Louise Hornbacher in *An Everyday Guide To Your Health*. "Breathing itself dramatizes and actualizes the essential polarities of life: inspiration/ expiration, expansion/contraction, tension/relaxation, positive/ negative, external/internal, giving/receiving. Each breath represents a cycle of birth and death, in the delicate balance of which lies life itself. Each inhalation can be an inspiration, an opening, a receiving, a welcoming of the world. And each outbreath can be a returning, a giving, a releasing of the world. So allow yourself to be breathed."

Breathing cannot be learned without proper alignment of the body. Judith H. Lasaters, a regular contributor to the *Yoga Journal* writes, "Since the ribs are encasing the lungs, attached to the spinal column, it is of crucial importance that you learn to sit or lie down where you would have the maximum freedom for the lungs."

"Because sitting upright is often a challenge to one's attention," as Arthur Kilmurray states in the March/April 1983 issue of the *Yoga Journal*, I recommend a supine position at first to avoid the problem of slouching. Kilmurray continues: "You may focus totally on the breathing process; the sitting can be practiced separately. Later, as breathing and sitting both become more natural, they may be combined."

Please refer to section V, chapter 3 on Daily Living Habits and read Corrective Sleeping Habits, so you will know how to properly place yourself on the floor. These simple, easy-to-follow innovative positions have helped many of my students who have breathing problems such as asthma, emphysema, cystic fibrosis, high and low blood pressure, cerebral palsy, cardial and pulmonary dysfunctions, scoliosis, arthritis, and multiple sclerosis.

My heart goes out to people who are made to feel all the more limited because their breathing inadequacies have been diagnosed. Usually, they are given only two alternatives: to slow down or rely on the crutch of their medical inhalators, which cannot leave their sides. As a last resort, these people come to me to find out in only an hour that there is hope; they can gain control of their breath. Every week I hear, "If only someone had told me this years ago." This section on breathing is my attempt to reach many more of these people than I can at my studio. Please share this information with any family members or friends who might feel an exercise book is beyond them because of their breathing difficulties.

Now that you have a mental picture of how the breathing process goes, read and practice the breathing exercises. By following them with your new corrective exercise program, you will find many new and attractive qualities and resources. Breathing correctly gives you many wide-ranging rewards: your skin will glow, your energy level will be more vital, your movements more rhythmical, your heart stronger, and your voice clearer and more pleasing to the ear.

With all these good pointers, let's move along to find a position that's the most comfortable for you and that will help you maintain an aligned and balanced body—free to breathe!

POSITIONS TO AID IN PROPER BREATHING

Supine Technique

1. Lie on your back. Take your hands to tuck your buttocks downward, placing the sacrum flat on the floor. Inhale and use your elbows to lift up your chest. Exhale. Squeeze the shoulder blades together and lower them to the floor. Elongate the back of the neck and place your head so the face is looking straight up, as in figure 1. Review section V, chapter 3 on Daily Living Habits and read Corrective Sleeping Habits.

2. Place a firmly rolled-up towel under your lower ribs, as in figure 2. This lifts the rib cage and allows the lower lumbar spine to extend.

3. Place a facecloth, folded in half and firmly rolled up, between the shoulder blades going lengthwise with the spine, as in figure 3. This opens the chest and relaxes the neck. When inhaling, lift slightly upward. Upon exhaling, squeeze the shoulder blades downward around the facecloth until it's comfortable.

4. Place a folded blanket lengthwise under the spine. Extend it from the top of the head to the top of the sacrum; the coccyx rests evenly on the floor. Make sure you don't pinch in the lower back. Tuck your buttocks down and out of the way, as in figure 4. This position helps to open the rib cage and awakens the spinal intelligence.

5. If your pubic bone is lower than your hipbones, when you lie down, fold a beach towel in half and roll it firmly, placing it high under the thighs, as in figure 5. This keeps the pelvic girdle aligned. Make sure your pelvic triangle is level.

6. Roll a towel to fit comfortably under the neck, as in figure 6. This gives support to the neck and aligns the head. If the chin ever lifts up in any of the above positions, fold a towel to support the head so that the chin is parallel to or very slightly dropped toward the floor.

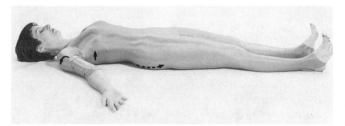

Figure 1

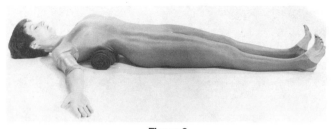

Figure 2

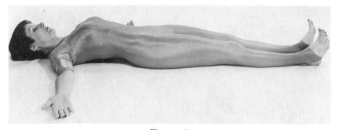

Figure 3

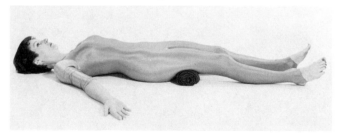

Figure 4

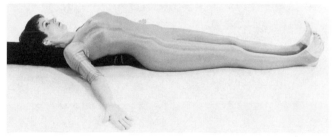

Figure 5

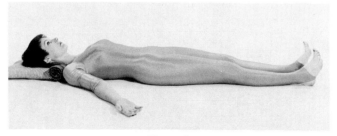

Figure 6

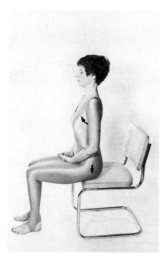

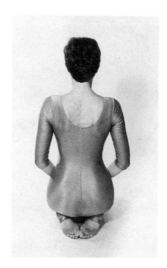

| Figure 1 | Figure 2 |

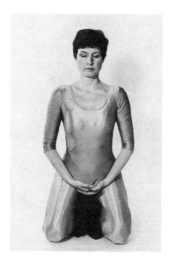

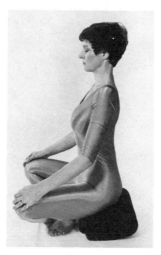

| Figure 3 | Figure 4 |

Sitting Technique

1. Sit at the edge of a chair or bench with a flat, firm base. Place your heels directly under your knees. Sit straight up on your ischial bones (sit bones), as in figure 1. Do not slouch. This position aligns and balances the body. Do not sit back into the chair; use the support system you have been given.

2. Sit in a high-heeled position, where your heels are drawn toward each other and under each ischium bone, as in figure 2. This helps in keeping the pelvic girdle aligned and the back relaxed.

3. For those who can't sit as in figure 2, sit on a rolled-up blanket, as in figure 3. Use as many blankets as you need to relieve the pressure on the ankles and knees.

4. Sit in a Lotus or simple cross-legged position. Whatever the position, do not allow the knees to be above the hip joints. Use as many folded blankets as you need to make this comfortable, as in figure 4. Keep the pelvis perpendicular to the floor. This releases the spine upward, maintains the normal spinal curves, and distributes the weight evenly across the sit bones.

COMPLETE BREATH OR RIB CAGE BREATHING

It is important to allow the Complete or Rib Cage Breath to flow in a slow, smooth, fluid, continuous rhythm. In executing the breath while exercising, the rate of breathing should adjust to the effort. The larger the effort, the more necessary it is to exhale completely; release tension; and breathe in a deep, full breath to gain the energy you need.

Once you learn the correct way of breathing, begin the day with some deep, slow breaths while lying in bed, before you get up. Take advantage of every chance to be outdoors. During the day, at work or elsewhere, remember to take time for some deep Rib Cage Breaths. When you practice your exercises, remember to synchronize the timing of your deep breaths in rhythm with the motion of your body. At the end of the evening take a few moments for a short session of breathing in bed. You will probably fall right to sleep.

Taking time to assimilate short but frequent sessions during the day will let Rib Cage Breathing become a habit. You will soon find yourself breathing the correct way most of the time. Complete Breathing will produce a healthier and cleaner body, a clearer and calmer mind, and a heightened spirit.

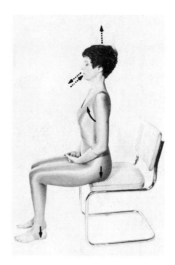

Figure 1

Props

A chair or bench with a flat, firm surface.

Body Placement

Sit on the edge of the chair with your head straight up, balancing on your ischial bones. Put your heels directly under your knees, as in figure 1.

Technique

1. Sit with a straight spine.
2. Concentrate on the back floor of the throat, as in figure 2.
3. With mouth w-i-d-e open and the back floor of the throat open, start to breathe in and out with long, slow breaths. You are concentrating on where you would gargle. Continue to practice this until you feel the air pass through the throat. It's as if you are "tasting" the breath. This means you have found the correct spot.
4. Before you close your lips, it is helpful to envision the air entering through your ears, not through your nose. I say this because the nose should stay relaxed with no sensation. You do not actually breathe through your ears, of course, but it sure sounds and feels like it.
5. With your mouth still open, as if using a suction pump, begin to draw in the air from the back floor of the throat. When you feel that taste of air, close your lips, keep the throat open, and continue to breathe. Think ears *not* nose.

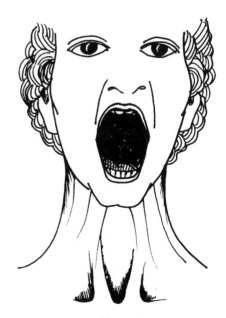

Figure 2

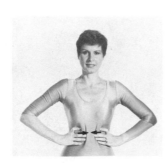

Figure 4

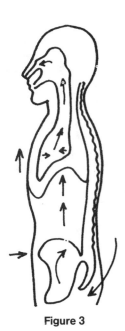

Figure 3

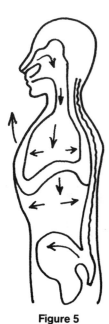

Figure 5

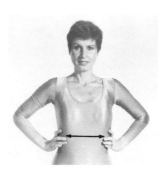

Figure 6

Figure 7

6. To work it from a closed mouth, arrange the inside of your mouth and throat so that the tip of the tongue presses lightly against the back of the upper front teeth. Drop down your tongue so that the throat is open, as if you were stifling a yawn.

7. Now that you have the technique of how to keep the passageway open for the breath, let's follow it down through the body.

8. Ready! Exhale to the count of eight, contracting the abdomen and rib cage. Keep the chest up and open, as in figure 3. You can place your hand on the side of your ribs, with the thumb toward the back, as in figure 4. Apply pressure with the palm of your hands to feel the action.

9. Hold to the count of two. It should be a natural pause. Do not be tense.

10. Inhale to the count of four, relaxing the rib cage and letting it expand outward—not up in front, but out from the sides and back, as in figures 5 and 6. To complete the inhalation, extend the sternum. This will completely fill the lungs.

11. Hold to the count of two. Keep it a natural pause. Repeat this breathing rhythm, as in figure 7. Work to have both the inhalation and exhalation flow in a slow, smooth, fluid rhythm. If the suggested rhythm of eight (exhale, hold to count of two, inhale to count of four) is not comfortable for you, work slowly at your own rate and gradually build up to it.

Tips

1. As you improve, there will be a need to increase gradually the duration of your inhalation, hold, and exhalation to a timing that is natural and complete for you.

2. Remember to blend these three stages of breathing so they will flow. No staccato!

3. Become sensitive to the movement of the abdomen, diaphragm, and rib cage.

4. Train the ears to monitor the sound of the breaths and pauses.

5. Throughout practice, the brain is kept passive but alert to monitor your time and posture and maintain an even breath rhythm.

Benefits

It is the most important physical and emotional exercise you can ever do for yourself.

PROCEDURES AND PRECAUTIONS

The next two exercises, the Sectional-Mudra and Alternate Breathing, are more advanced, so I recommend that you consider the following procedures and precautions. Don't be alarmed by the list or use it as an excuse to avoid learning to breathe correctly. The suggestions are intended to ensure that the experience be a pleasant and successful one!

1. Always practice in a well-ventilated room without drafts.
2. Wear loose, comfortable clothing.
3. Practice on a stomach that is empty of all except light liquids. Never practice vigorous breathing until an hour or two has elapsed after a light meal and two to three hours after a heavy meal.
4. Light food can be taken half an hour after finishing.
5. Before starting, the bowels and bladder should be emptied.
6. You must sit with the back absolutely erect and the complete spine perpendicular to the floor.
7. There should be no strain felt in the facial muscles, eyes, ears, neck, shoulders, or arms. If you are in the Lotus position, deliberately relax the legs and feet.
8. Eyes should be closed to encourage proper moisture and to discourage a dry, burning sensation in the eyes.
9. Throughout practice, the brain is kept passive but alert. The ear listens for the proper sound of the breath. In Mudra Breathing, the hand is used to control the breath flow.
10. The student must be alert and sensitive to the flow of breath within him or herself, while being conscious of time, posture, and maintaining an even breath rhythm.
11. Each student should measure his or her own capacity and not exceed it. Capacity is reached when the smooth rhythm of breathing is lost.
12. Do not overdo it. These breathing exercises are not complicated. However, they are very concentrated; so be careful. After any controlled breathing, always have a period in your relaxed natural rhythm to stabilize yourself.

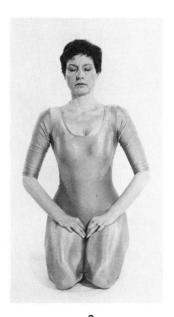

a

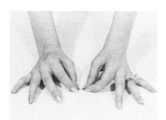

b

Figure 1

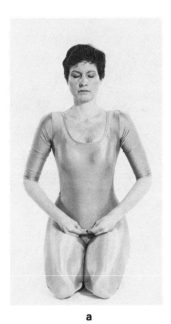

a

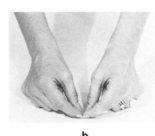

b

Figure 2

SECTIONAL-MUDRA BREATH

The Sectional-Mudra Breath aids breathing into restricted areas and activates each area to its fullest capacity.

A mudra (symbol) usually refers to a ritual gesture of the fingers and hands. Many mudras induce calmness by affecting certain nerves. Ancient Hindu treatises minutely classify the nodis (72,000 vital energy passages in the body), which loosely correspond to the nerve passages, and show their relationship with the mind. The mudra process brings air into specific areas of the lungs while restricting other centers.

Props

None

Body Placement

Sit in the high-heel sitting position with the heels of the hands on top of the thighs at the crease where the legs connect with the torso. Lean forward very slightly so that there is a mild pressure on the peripheral nerve on the top of the thigh, as in figure 1a.

Technique

1. Remember, the diaphragm and abdomen are located up inside your lower ribs, not in your belly.
2. To fill the lower lobes of the lungs (Diaphragmatic Breathing), connect the thumb and index finger of each hand and stretch the other three fingers, as in figure 1b.
3. Exhale fully. Then inhale, feeling where the air goes without mentally directing it. (Mental direction can interfere with the mudra.) You will find the lower lobes filling.
4. Repeat five times.
5. To fill the middle lobes (Intercostal Breathing), keep the thumb and index finger joined, but tuck the other fingers under into the cushions of the palms, as in figures 2a and b.
6. Exhale fully to empty all lobes. Then, without mental direction, as before, inhale and feel the air, which will now flow into the middle lobes of the lungs.
7. Repeat five times.

8. To fill the upper lobes (Clavicular Breathing), the thumb is tucked into the center of the palm, and the four fingers are wrapped around it, as in figures 3a and b.

9. Exhale fully. Inhale until the upper lungs are comfortably but fully expanded.

10. Repeat five times.

Variation

1. The mudra for the full Complete Breath is with the knuckles together, nails facing upward, and the little finger sides of the hands touching the abdomen just above the navel, as in figures 4a and b. With this gesture, the Complete Breath automatically takes over.

2. Exhale fully. Inhale with the Complete Breath as you feel all three lobes filling up. Don't cut off your breath; extend it as long as you can. You will be surprised at how much you can take in.

3. To exhale, reverse the process and make sure you exhale long enough to empty all the stale air.

4. Repeat ten or more times.

Tips

1. The mudra for the full Complete Breath can be used in any sitting or lying position, and the appropriate sections of the lungs will fill.

2. However, to affect the lower, middle, and upper lobes, a sitting posture must be applied. To restrict the separate sections, pressure must be kept on the peripheral nerve in the crease of the thigh.

3. To prove the efficacy of these mudras, make the upper lung mudra with one hand and the lower with the other. Exhale fully and then breathe. It will feel as though one shoulder is being lifted up, or that only one side of the body is working.

Benefits

The Sectional-Mudra Breath aids breathing into the restricted areas and activates the other areas to their fullest capacity.

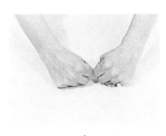

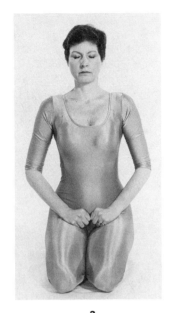

b

a

Figure 3

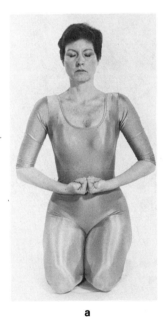

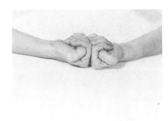

b

a

Figure 4

ALTERNATE BREATHING

Alternate Breathing consists of the Complete Rib Cage Breath, but emphasizes a deep controlled breath through one nostril at a time to bring purification of the nerves. It usually is practiced after the exercise routine or just before relaxation and is a vital part of the Yoga practice. When we do this exercise, we are to concentrate on exhaling completely, letting out all the carbon dioxide. When we inhale, we replenish our body with a flow of fresh oxygen, which we hold for awhile to allow for absorption into the system.

Props

None

Body Placement

1. Sit up with a straight back in one of the mentioned sitting positions that are comfortable for you.
2. The finger placement can be your choice. In figure 1, the index and middle fingers are turned down so the thumb and ring finger are close to the nose, with the little finger next to the ring finger. In figure 2, both fingers are placed on the space between the eyebrows, leaving the other fingers free to close the nose.

Technique

1. Sit with an erect spine and close your eyes.
2. Completely exhale from both nostrils.
3. Close the right nostril with the right thumb.
4. Draw in the air very slowly through the left nostril.
5. Close the left nostril with the ring and little fingers of the right hand. (Both nostrils are now closed.)
6. Pause. Remove your thumb and exhale slowly through the right nostril.
7. Inhale slowly through the same side (right nostril).
8. Close both nostrils and pause.
9. Remove your ring and little fingers and exhale slowly through the left nostril.
10. This process of inhalation, hold, and exhalation, constitutes one round. Start with five rounds and gradually increase the number to ten rounds.

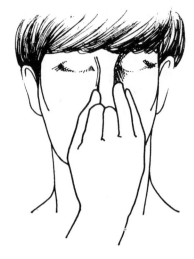

Figure 1

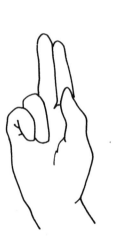

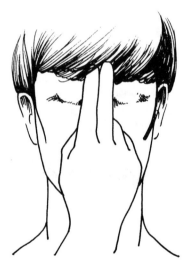

Figure 2

Variations

1. Begin with equal counts of breathing in and out rhythmically. Start from 5 counts and work to 8 counts. This is called the "purifying breath."

2. If you have practiced the purifying breath for awhile and feel comfortable in it, you may increase your exhalation count and inhale 5 counts-pause-and work up to exhaling to 10 counts. Advance only if you can maintain a smooth rhythm.

3. After you achieve mastery over the 5-pause-10 counts, you may apply a retention (hold) between breaths. Start from a count of: inhale-hold the breath in for 5 counts-exhale for 10 counts and work gradually to 5-20-10. It is not necessary to carry this further. The count should be increased only as long as it is comforable.

4. This precision is achieved only after long practice. Do not attempt it all at once.

5. Only experienced students, after inhalation, may apply a contraction of the anal sphincter muscle, which pulls up the lower abdomen toward the diaphragm.

6. Do not attempt to hold your breath after exhalation until you have mastered the 5-20-10 count. Make sure you are under the guidance of an experienced teacher.

7. When done correctly and with caution, Alternate Breathing exercises are beneficial in soothing frayed nerves and bring about a sense of tranquility.

Tips

1. Persons suffering from angina pectoris (a symptom of heart disease characterized by sharp pains in the chest) have found marked improvement from deep breathing through alternate nostrils. This procedure is recommended by heart specialists.

2. Persons suffering from high blood pressure or heart trouble should never attempt to hold their breath in after an inhalation. They can practice Alternate Breathing without the retention and gain beneficial effects.

3. Persons suffering from low blood pressure can do Alternate Breathing with retention *only* after inhalation for beneficial effects. They should not retain the breath after exhalation.

Benefits

Alternate Breathing is the key to mental and physical well-being. It can stabilize our moods.

2. Proper Body Alignment

What is "good" posture? Many times we were told or ordered by parents, gym teachers, or drill sergeants to: Stand up straight! Suck in your stomach! Throw the shoulders back! Sit up Straight! You probably endured this as many times as I and with the same results—an attempt at perfection that left you uncomfortable in much of your body. Most likely you were tense in your lower back, which you arched to support the upper body in this unnatural position. In my own personal search for the elusive ideal of perfectly balanced posture, I discovered that the place to begin to align the body is not from the top but from the feet.

Go to a mirror and stand sideways. There should be an imaginary straight line from the center of the ankle, knee, hip, shoulder, and ear. (The ear is off because you are turning your head to see.) Now look at your bare feet. Do you grip with your toes? Is the weight leaning forward into the front of the foot? Do your feet roll in or out? Do you feel any pressure in the small of the back, knees, hip, or neck? If you do not line up with that imaginary plumb line, then you are out of alignment and have "bad" posture, which can result in back, hip, or neck pain. You will come back to the mirror a little later.

For all the problems it causes, the human spine is actually an engineering marvel that serves far more complex and versatile roles than any structure yet devised by humankind. Gravity constantly pulls the body down so that muscles supporting the vertebrae must work to keep the spine from collapsing. As Arthur Kilmurray observed in the March 1983 issue of the *Yoga Journal*, the spine must "carry the weight of the human frame; be flexible; allow bending and rotation in all directions, even under heavy loads; be hollow to allow delicate nerves and blood vessels to pass through it; and emerge from its sides without being damaged during movement. All that, and function adequately for a lifetime."

I visualize the spinal column, roughly speaking, as three "cubes" balanced above two pillars (legs). They are the 1) pelvic girdle, 2) shoulder girdle and thorax, and 3) head. They are connected by two "linkages," the neck and lumbar spine. If one's body is not aligned correctly, it is a difficult balancing act for the spine and joints to carry. Two common stress areas are between the atlas and axis cervical vertebrae, and the fifth lumbar vertebrae, where the lumbar spine connects with the sacrum.

The linkages should be balanced and free (in neutral) not too far forward nor backward, but in the center. They should be properly aligned and supporting the three cubes. Because the spine is responsible for balance and support as well as flexibility, the vertebrae must be supported in the way a tree can be supported by stakes and guy wires. The guy wires are our muscles.

The *pelvic girdle* forms the base for the spinal column. If the pelvis is off balance, it will affect the position of the lower back (lower linkage). The proper pelvic alignment is controlled by the muscles of the hips and abdomen.

If the upper part of the pelvis rotates forward and downward, the forward curve (lordosis) increases in the lumbar vertebrae. The spine "falls" forward toward the abdomen, and the result is swayback (excessive lumbar lordosis). Because the abdominal muscles attach to the upper part of the pelvis, weakness of these muscles is a major cause of this condition. Also, because the gluteal muscles in the buttocks attach to the back of the lower pelvis, weakness of these muscles also contributes to this forward rotation.

The psoas muscle, which attaches on the inside of the lumbar, traverses over the pelvic basin and attaches to the upper inside section of the thighbone. It is crucial in determining the amount of tilt the pelvis takes. A tight psoas muscle tends to pull the lumbar spine toward the groin. The lower back and the groin area are stressed by a short, tight psoas and eventually will distort out of their proper position, causing a swayback condition and an excessive protruding belly. Swayback causes the muscles, ligaments, and other tissues of the back to become shortened and tight and results in pain, even though there has been no exertion or injury. Furthermore, an exertion or sudden movement is now an invitation to even greater pain.

The *shoulder girdle* and *thorax* should have a lifting sensation so as not to hang down into the waist, which puts a lot of pressure on the vulnerable lower back. The rib cage houses the lungs and with the correct alignment can give them a better opportunity to function to their fullest capacity.

The *head* weighs about fifteen pounds, which is a lot of weight for the delicate cervical spine (top link) to carry. The neck and head balance on top of the shoulder girdle and are at the mercy of the proper support of the shoulder blades.

Keep the cubes and links in mind when you read the basic principles of application for each main body area in section IV.

It has been estimated that up to of eight million Americans are suffering the torment of back pain, whether induced by athletic zeal, hard work, pregnancy, or simply the toll of aging. Approximately 85 percent of back pain is now attributed to muscular weakness or imbalance.

In the vast majority of individuals with low back pain, the underlying problem is mechanical. There is improper postural alignment with a weakness of certain muscles. Other muscles and ligaments are tight and short. In such individuals a proper back exercise and postural correction program almost always results in the relief of symptoms. Even if there is an underlying problem such as disc degeneration or arthritic changes, symptoms can almost completely disappear.

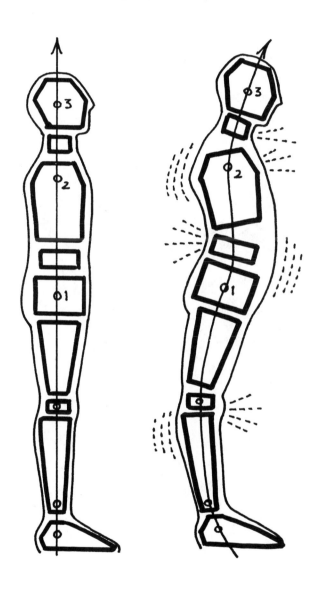

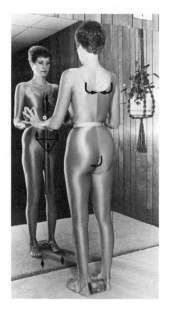

Figure 1

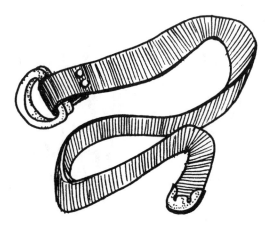

Figure 2

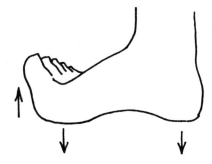

Figure 3

Although the Bodysense Method might seem simple, it is an amazingly effective exercise and postural correction program that will help almost all patients with back problems. The simple and nonstrenuous exercises are specifically designed to strengthen key muscles, stretch out tightness in the low back, and restore normal postural alignment of the low back and pelvis. Once this has been accomplished and symptoms have been relieved, the correct posture must be maintained, or symptoms will recur in the future. One must learn to sit, lie, stand, walk, and carry out all of the normal activities of daily living with the low back and pelvis in the correct postural position.

Read section V, chapter 3 on Daily Living Habits for more details.

BUILDING BLOCKS OF POSTURE

Props

1. Put a tape down the middle of your mirror.
2. Tie a 2½-foot pole or a vacuum attachment to the front of your body, using a nylon belt with two rings to slide closed, as in figure 2. I want the pole pulled very tight against the body.
3. You might feel a little suffocated until you align your body.
4. Place a block (tomato can) between your heels—not near the arches, but at the back end of the heels.

Body Placement

1. Stand in front of the mirror with the pole very tight and the block between your heels, as in figure 1.
2. Place your fingers on the mirror at rib level.
3. To align the pelvic triangle, exhale as you contract the navel inward, drawing the pubic bone forward to the pole.
4. Inhale, elongate up out of your waist, drawing the sternum (chest bone) forward to the pole.
5. The pole will become more comfortable as you work through the next eight steps to "line up" your Building Blocks of Posture.

Technique

1. Raise all of your toes, while pressing the balls of your feet into the floor. The weight should be evenly distributed between the heels and balls of your feet, as in figure 3. Work as if you are aligning four tires under your feet. The block should help to align the ankles and balance the arches.

2. Now that your feet are based correctly, look at your knees. Are they hyperextended, knock-kneed, bowed, or crossed, as in figure 4?

3. If your knees are knock-kneed, bowed, or crossed, raise the kneecaps, tighten your buttocks as you rotate the thighs, bringing the knees to face straight forward. For hyperextended knees, ease the knees by bending them slightly, then raise the kneecaps. If you are not in these categories, raise your kneecaps without the rotation.

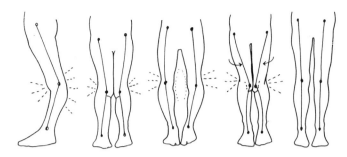

Figure 4

4. To continue aligning the body, exhale and contract your abdomen as you further tuck the tailbone downward and inward, while pressing the pubic bone to the pole. Lessen the arch in your back. Then, inhale and elongate your rib cage, pulling it up out of your waist. Align the sternum to the pole, as in figure 5. (I use the phrases "press the pubic bone to the pole" and "the tailbone draws the pubic bone forward" because so many people carry the pubic bone way behind of where it should be [swayback]. Ideally, in its neutral, aligned position, it seats less than a quarter of an inch behind the frontal hipbone.) If the pole is pressing too hard, back off a little; you don't need to work this strenuously.

5. Exhale, as you feel the pelvis come into balance. Inhale and concentrate on elongating upward from the waist, elevate the rib cage, and extend the sternum (breastbone). Do *not* thrust the chest forward. The pole will help to keep you in line.

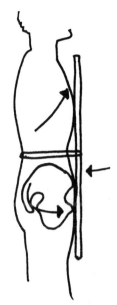

Figure 5

6. Now rotate your shoulders in a backward and downward movement toward the middle of the back. Bring the shoulder blades toward each other, as in figure 6. Exhale. This example is for rounded shoulders (sunken chest syndrome) and not for those with good or military posture.

7. To complete the alignment, keep the back of the neck lengthened. To attain this, try to touch an imaginary hand held one inch above your head.

8. The weight of your entire body column should be equally distributed between the heels and balls of your feet. When you have attained this, relax your toes and buttocks; but do not lose the lift you feel throughout your body. Take the pole off and see what a help it was to you. You may feel some discomfort from your new placement if you have been out of line for a long period of time. It will help you to concentrate on *elongating as you inhale and working into balance as you exhale*. With continued effort from this stable foundation, your spine can be lengthened not only by muscular effort but by sensing Bodysense as well. "Thinking tall" can become a reality!

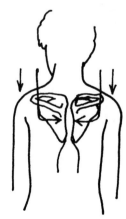

Figure 6

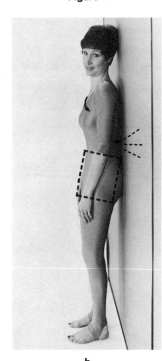

Figure 1

Figure 2
Incorrect

USING A CORNER OR DOORWAY TO ALIGN THE SPINE

Props

1. Choose an outer corner where two walls meet or the edge of a doorway.

Body Placement

1. With your back against the corner, stand with the heels four inches away from the edge and the toes raised.
2. Rest the sacrum and the back of the head against the edge.
3. Place your fingers in the small of the back, as in figure 1.
4. There should remain a gap of about one inch between the lumbar spine and the corner. Study the incorrect positions in figure 2, to know what you should not look like.
5. You will find your waist in varying degrees from the corner, but the pelvic cube triangle should be balanced at all times.
6. The purpose of this exercise is to attain the natural curve of the lumbar spine, which is about one inch from the corner.

Technique

1. Bend your knees to slide down the corner, as in figure 3.
2. Use your hands to tuck your buttocks downward. Press the sacrum (boney area above the tailbone), *not* your waist, on the wall, as in figure 3a.
3. With the elbows bent and behind the ribs, inhale and lift the ribs *up* (not forward) out of the waist, as in figure 3b.
4. While exhaling, roll the shoulders back and down, and apply a blade squeeze.
5. Inhale and elongate the upper body with only the back of the head and sacrum touching the wall. Men might find this hard to do because of their shoulder development.
6. While exhaling, rotate the pelvis so the two frontal hipbones

move up toward the ribs, while the coccyx (tailbone) moves down and forward toward the pubic bone. The pubic bone and frontal hipbone form a vertical triangle.

7. Inhale and start to slide up the wall with only your sacrum and head touching (not your waist), as in figure 4a.
8. Exhale and continue to slide up. If you find you are losing your vertical triangle (pelvic tuck), don't tighten your legs—keep them slightly bent.
9. Inhale and elongate. Exhale as you maintain a contracted abdomen and rotated pelvis tuck. Come away from the corner, as in figure 4b.
10. You should be standing perfectly aligned on your own two feet. Feel the balance!
11. Repeat five times.

Tips

1. If it is difficult for you to balance with your heels four inches away from the edge, you may move further away to attain a balance. But keep your waist one inch from the corner.
2. Keep practicing this exercise to attain the correct rotation for your individual alignment.
3. The legs should never lock back; they should work to be straight.
4. It is beneficial to do this several times a day.
5. If you have a narrow doorway, apply Technique steps 1-10 with your back against the doorway and press both hands against the opposite side, as in figures 5a and b.

Benefits

The back and pelvic girdle are aligned and strengthened. The abdominals are working correctly, relieving low back pressure.

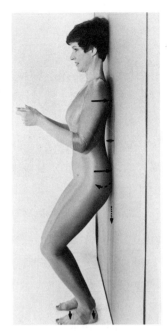 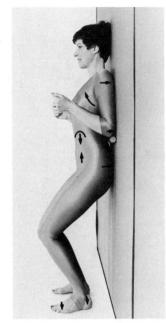

a   **Figure 3**   b

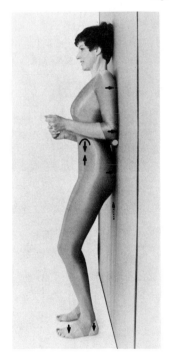 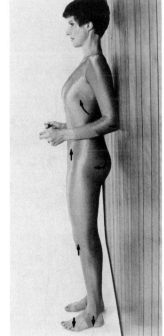

a   b

Figure 4

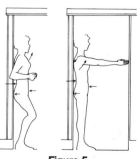

a   b

Figure 5

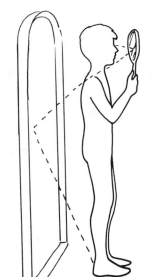
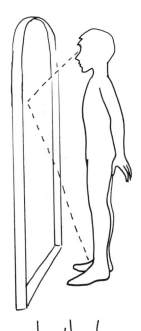

MIRROR TEST

1. Feet

When standing, the feet should always be grounded; that is, firmly planted on the floor with a lifted arch and centered ankle. Be aware of the four tires on each foot; make sure they are aligned and that you are balancing between the balls of the feet and heels, with the toes up or extended. Don't grip with your toes. Your feet should feel light, lifted, and sensitive, yet deeply grounded. Even when the feet are not weight bearing, you should maintain the same alignment. For more details on the feet, read section IV, chapter 1.

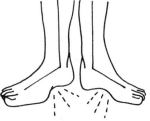
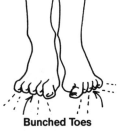

Outward Turn

Bunched Toes

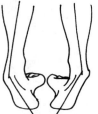

Rolled-Out Ankles (Varus)

Rolled-In Ankles (Valgus)

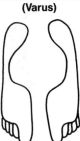
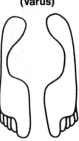
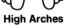

High Arches

INCORRECT

Flat Feet

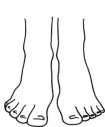
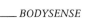

Neutral

CORRECT

2. Knees

The knee joints are complex not only because of crossing ligaments and vulnerable cartilage, but also because they support weight.

The kneecaps should always face forward. When doing standing exercises, the knee should be lifting up toward the thigh. Even when the knee is going to be bent, you lift the kneecap upward to protect and gain proper control of the knee. Be careful! I mean a lifted kneecap, not a knee pushed backward to make it tight; this is hyperextending the knee. Your knee should be straight with a toned, lifted feeling. See section IV, chapter 1.

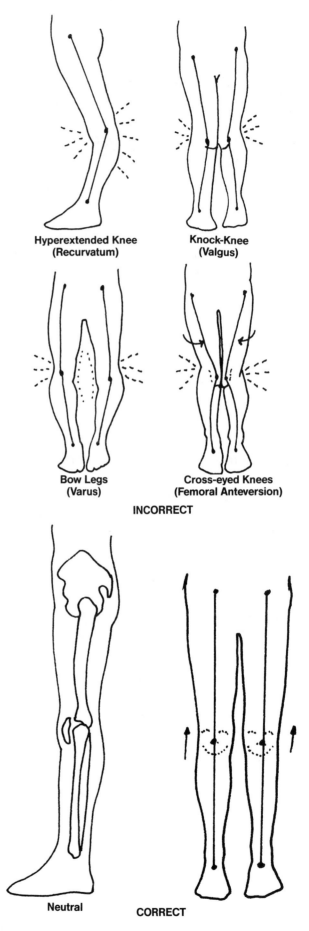

Hyperextended Knee
(Recurvatum)

Knock-Knee
(Valgus)

Bow Legs
(Varus)

Cross-eyed Knees
(Femoral Anteversion)

INCORRECT

Neutral

CORRECT

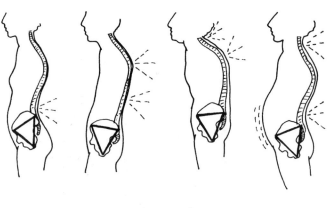

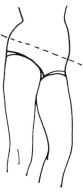

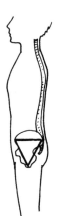

INCORRECT

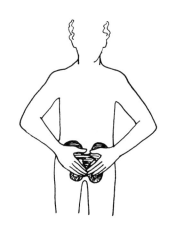

CORRECT

3. Pelvic Girdle

The pelvic girdle is composed of three joints: 1) the hip joint, 2) the sacroiliac joint, and 3) the pubic symphysis, all of which work in unison to provide mobility and stability for the body. The ball-and-socket configuration of the hip is designed particularly to allow great mobility and stability. The pelvis can assume three positions. As you stand, the correct one is the neutral position in which the pelvis is vertical and the ischial bones point straight down to the floor. Place your fingers on the pubic bone and the heels of your hands on the frontal hipbones to form a triangle. To produce the effect we want, imagine keeping a dime between your buttocks. Now squeeze your buttocks, drawing the dime upward. If you are standing up, the tailbone tucks downward and forward, pushing the pubic bone in line with the frontal hipbones. This forms a balanced vertical pelvic triangle with the waistline completely horizontal.

When lying down, the pelvic triangle should be horizontal, balancing on the sacrum.

When sitting, the pelvic triangle is vertical, balancing straight up on the ischial bones. Once the pelvis is in a vertical position, action has to be brought in to the sacroiliac joints to keep the two frontal hipbones vertically above the groin.

When working with the pelvic girdle, remember to maintain a squaring-off application to each exercise. You should not have a rounded, locked feeling. Read section IV, chapter 3.

4. The Spinal Column

The pelvis is a bowl-like construction at the lower end of the spinal column that can rock forward and backward. When out of alignment, the pelvis places unnecessary pressure in the lumbar spine and, if not corrected, the pressure travels up into the neck.

The lumbar spine acts as a linkage between the pelvic girdle and shoulder girdle. It should always remain free and balanced, with no pressure, even while doing bends.

To stretch the back safely, it must first be positioned correctly. In bent-over positions, the entire trunk must be straight so the spine moves as one unit. There should remain a gentle groove (not a bumpy path) up through the back, the spine being recessed. It is important that the groove appear or feel balanced to the touch. I don't want any deep gullies! The same groove is true for the supine position. You automatically use the correct position when you balance your pelvic triangle horizontally and use a pole at the waist. Read section IV, chapter 5.

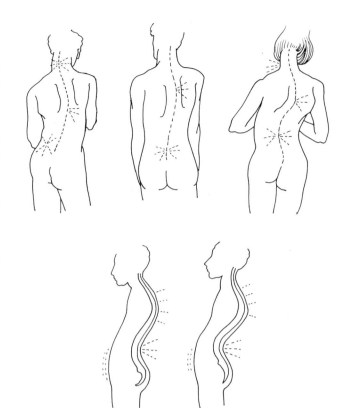

INCORRECT

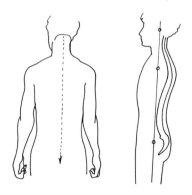

CORRECT

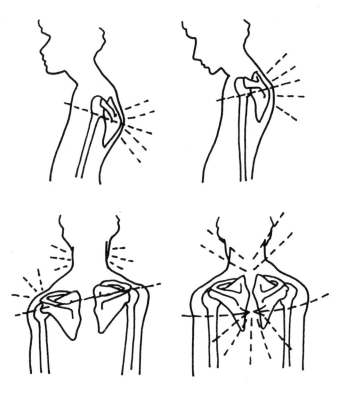

INCORRECT

CORRECT

5. Shoulder Girdle

A weak upper body taxes the lower back by making it work harder to carry and balance a full trunk.

Does your chest sink in when you stand? To align the upper body, clasp your hands behind you. Inhale and extend your chest up and frontward. While exhaling, rotate your arms to squeeze the shoulder blades together. Repeat four times. Let go of your hands. You now should be standing much more erect and balanced over the pelvic girdle. Feel the lightness. When you tuck under the tailbone, you eliminate pressure in the lower lumbar.

Are your shoulders rolled up and the blades pointed into the floor when you lie down? To align yourself, use your elbows to lift the chest, and before you lower, squeeze the blades together, landing flat on the blades. The shoulders should be rotating toward the floor, and the shoulder girdle should be evenly open in front and back and top and bottom. When lying down, the chest is completely horizontal. When standing, the chest is vertical. For correct alignment your chest should *never* be slanted. Read section IV, chapter 6.

6. Neck and Head

The neck acts as a linkage where the nerve cords of the brain pass through to the spinal canal. It is very important to create and maintain space between the cervical vertebrae so that the nerves have more freedom to function smoothly.

Most people let their head hang forward or reach with their chin while doing exercises, which puts tremendous pressure in the neck.

I always remind my students to keep their head elongated and balanced, the way it grows. The position of the head should balance as an extension of the spine. You don't *put* the head into position; it remains free as it balances above the proper alignment of the shoulder girdle.

When you lie down, your head should be balanced on the center back of the head, with the face positioned straight upward. The chin should not be tilted upward or downward. If needed, fold a towel the correct thickness to make the head level and to relax the neck. Read section IV, chapter 6 on Corrective Sleeping Habits for the Neck.

If your head leans forward of the torso when you stand, align your head by drawing it back, as a cobra would. You will feel relief in the neck, and the shoulders can sit as the foundation for the neck and head.

The neck should be relaxed while doing all your exercises (except, of course, neck exercises). The head should follow the alignment of the shoulders to keep the neck free and to allow the nerves to function smoothly.

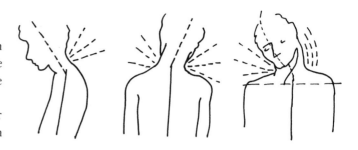

INCORRECT

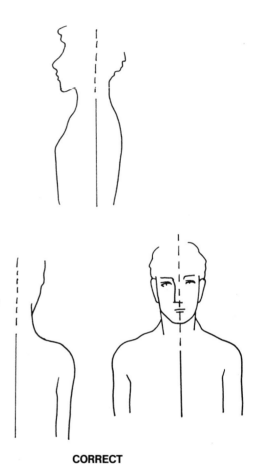

CORRECT

Section IV

Targeted Exercises

1. *Feet, Ankles, and Knees*
2. *Hamstrings, Thighs, Buttocks, and Groin*
3. *Hips and Pelvic Girdle*
4. *Abdominal Muscles*
5. *The Back*
6. *Chest, Shoulder Girdle, Neck, and Eyes*
7. *Elbows, Wrists, and Hands*

1. Feet, Ankles, and Knees

Eighty-seven percent of Americans have foot problems. Podiatrists know that the aching feet they see represent only a small amount of a large occurrence of pain and avoidable deformity. The United States Public Health Service's survey, as presented in the *New York Times Magazine* (23 April 1978), showed that foot ailments are our third most disabling health problem, after heart disease and cancer. Afflicted Americans squander some $200 million a year on over-the-counter foot medications and appliances. It is squandering because such medications and devices do not get at the basic problem—poor body mechanics. And body mechanics begin with the foot.

Just as the development of modern architecture depended upon the principle of the simple arch, people's physical structures and well-being rest upon the arches of their feet. The bones in the arches are held in shape and are controlled by ligaments and muscles. If they are deformed or slack, the arches flatten, and problems begin, extending throughout the body.

Despite the importance of the foot, few of us spend much time and effort stregthening the ligaments and muscles of our feet to ensure the firm foundation of our bodies' vehicle. When you think of it, we pay more attention to the balance, alignment, and wear of the tires of our cars than we do to the proper care of our feet. Think, again, of the relationship between your feet and the construction of a car. Just as a car has four tires, so too does the foot: the ball of the foot (the two front tires) and the heel (the two back tires).

When standing, the feet should always be grounded, firmly planted on the floor with a lifted arch and centered ankles. The weight should be evenly distributed and balanced between the front (ball of the foot) and back tires (the heel). I try to make my students aware of the four tires of the foot so that they keep the tires aligned and parallel with the toes extended when walking, standing, and exercising. Perfect balance means the feet feel light, lifted, and sensitive, yet deeply grounded—no flat tires!

The Foot and Ankle Relationship

So often, I hear complaints of weak ankles when the problem actually emanates from the feet. People tend to not understand that all parts of the body are connected. They don't look at the alignment of their feet or at their knees for the culprit to the

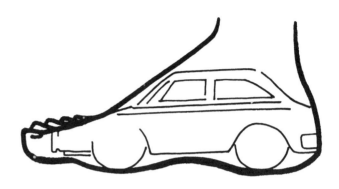

CORRECT

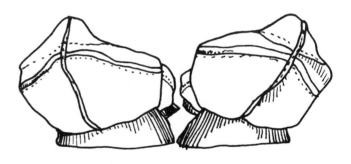

INCORRECT
Notice the Flat Tires in the Sneakers

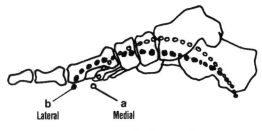

Longitudinal Arch

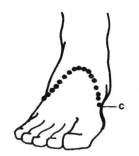

Transverse Metatarsal Arch

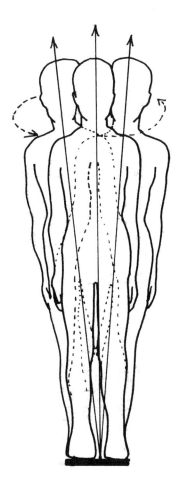

problem. Ida P. Rolf, in *rolfing: The Integration of Human Structures*, identifies three distinct arches in the foot, which balance the ankle and the knee. The spring action of the medial longitudinal arch (**a**) rides on top of the spring action of the lateral longitudinal arch (**b**). These transmit weight as well as distribute it. There is also a transverse metatarsal arch (**c**) that goes across the front of the foot. In any competent arch, contour is created and preserved not only by the configuration of the bones themselves but also by tough connective tissue that holds the two ends of the arch the way a bowstring that connects the ends of a bow. This allows the weight of the body to be spread as on the base of a triangle; but not all arches maintain their structural integrity. Some people are born with fallen arches or flat feet. Others develop these conditions because of inherent weaknesses in the muscles and injuries to their ligaments.

It is essential to strengthen the ligaments and muscles in our feet to help prevent and overcome foot deficiencies. The exercises in this chapter are designed to do just that. One of the first exercises I give my classes to heighten foot awareness is my "cone" experience.

Stand up and notice how your feet feel on the floor. How much of the foot is weight bearing? Now that you have made an evaluation of your feet, stand in perfect posture with your feet hip-width apart, hands at your side in military fashion, and eyes closed. It's as if you were in a cone with the feet being the base. Start tilting forward, without losing your balance; then tilt to the side, back, and other side, making a circle with your head. Keep your hips in a straight line. Make about ten slow rotations, and notice how your feet respond to the floor. Don't grip with your toes; extend them. Also, don't rotate from the hips; keep your body stiff. Draw a wide circle with your head. The width of your circle should be determined by the control of your balance.

Pause in the center, and repeat in the opposite direction for ten more rotations. At the end, pause in the center again, and before you open your eyes, take notice of your feet. How do they feel now? Deeper? Wider? Warmer? Open your eyes. This is what I call being grounded or submitting your feet to the floor. You should not, however, have to do this cone every time to ground yourself; you will be able to call upon your new-found feet awareness at will.

Dr. Rob Roy McGregor, a well-known sports podiatrist, writes, "Ninety percent of the knee problems can be managed by treatment of the feet." The foot is a much neglected, even an actively maligned part of the body. When it is not compelled to run several miles, jump up and down, or dance, it plods along humbly, bearing the weight of everything else. But when this delicate extremity is driven to reckless running or jumping, those little flaws of alignment, like the automobile with the poorly balanced wheels, can transmit bad vibrations upward. This jars things loose and grinds the knees, lower back, and parts as high up as the neck.

The Knees

If any of our body mechanics deviate greatly from proper alignment, then difficulties can appear even without the stress of sports or jogging. Proper posture starts from two parallel, aligned feet, standing firmly on their balanced four tires, then works its way up the leg to the knees. The knees should face straight ahead. Do not lock them back (hyperextended, as in figures 1a and c), but keep them eased and lifted upward (neutral, as in figures 1b and d). Lifting the knees upward (called making a face) stabilizes and secures the knee joint.

We owe a great deal to our knees. Without the knees' rubberband-like connectors, the tendons and ligaments, we couldn't move a muscle. Also, without the knees' cartilage and cushioning sacs, swinging into action would be something we could only contemplate; so we need to understand and protect our knees.

The knee joint is not only complex because of crossing ligaments and vulnerable cartilage, but it also supports the body's weight. Three other misalignments of the knee that break down the support system are knock-knees, bowlegs, and cross-eyed knees, as in figure 2.

The knee has been frequently referred to as "the unforgiving joint" because injury to it is often reflected long after the initial recovery. In sports, the knee is one of the most vulnerable joints. It acts as a hinge and a lever that glides, slides, and rotates. It is actually an unstable joint and depends on the soft tissue structures (muscles, tendons, ligaments, and cartilage) for its stability. The best anti-injury insurance is to exercise correctly with the feet and knees aligned.

Listen to your knees. When they hurt, *stop*. You are doing something wrong. Forget you ever heard "no pain, no gain." With the knee, it is *pain, no gain*. Remember, when walking, standing, or exercising, check to see that your feet are parallel; that the weight is between the balls and heels; and that the knees are eased, lifted, and in line with the feet.

The following exercises might seem too simple a solution for those of you in pain, but they work in the majority of cases. Those of you who will practice the Feet and Knee exercises and correct your walking and running habits will soon notice a tremendous reduction in feet and leg ailments. Some of my students have said their feet even look prettier.

The effort you put into the rehabilitation, alignment, and proper use of your feet, ankles, and knees will be of great value to you in the future. I am interested not only in how you function now, but also how you will function for years to come. Remember, when the feet and knees function improperly, they interfere with other functions of the body. Your feet are the foundation of your body; your body's function will be enhanced by what should be normal foot integrity. So, make each foot you put forward your best one!

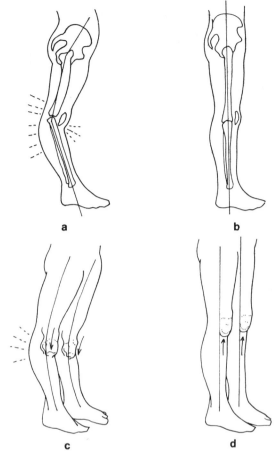

a

b

c

d

Figure 1

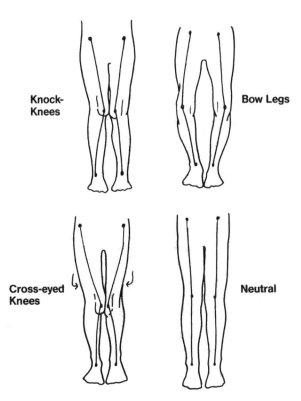

Knock-Knees

Bow Legs

Cross-eyed Knees

Neutral

Figure 2

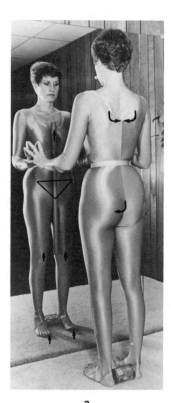

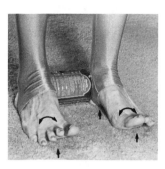

b

a

Figure 1

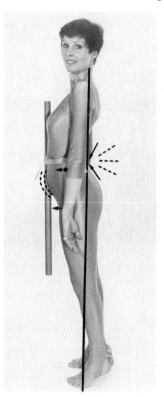

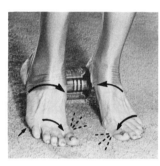

b

a

Figure 2
INCORRECT

FOOT, SHIN, AND KNEE STRENGTHENER

Props

1. A 2½-foot pole or the attachment from a vacuum cleaner.
2. A belt with double-ring loops.
3. A can of food, measuring 4½-inches tall.
4. A full-length mirror, as in figure 1a, or a small one that you can place on the floor.

Body Placement

1. Tie the pole *very* tightly around the waist.
2. Stand with your fingertips on the mirror and elbows bent by your ribs.
3. Place the can between the back part of your heels, as in figure 1b. Do *not* put it near the arches.

Technique

1. Start to inhale as you raise your toes and keep the balls of the feet on the floor. Continue inhaling while elongating your body up the pole.
2. Push lightly with the fingers and create a blade squeeze. While exhaling, keep the elongation as you contract the abdomen away from the pole and rotate the pubic bone to the pole. This balances the pelvic triangle, as in figure 1a.
3. Repeat five times to align your posture.
4. Look into the mirror, as in figure 1a, and make sure your feet are parallel with the heels hugging the can, as in figure 1b.
5. While inhaling, elongate up the pole. Make sure the sternum and pubic bone touch and the toes are still raised.
6. While exhaling, contract the abdomen. Keep the pubic bone to the pole and the knees facing forward. (If they don't, turn them.) Raise the heels and, while squeezing the can, balance

on the balls of your feet, as in figure 4. Study figures 2 and 3 for what *not* to do. Align the balls of both feet as if they were the four front tires of two cars, with the feet being in position to drive straight ahead.

7. Stay up for two more breaths, repeating Technique steps 4 and 5. You may have to lean forward to get up at first, as in figure 3, but do *not* lean and lose your alignment, as in figure 2. Bring yourself straight up in this position, aligning and balancing your body over the balls of the feet, as in figure 4.

8. Come down. You were a good sport to put up with the pole and can! Although they are uncomfortable at first, they really are necessary to teach you what needs to be aligned. Aren't they?

9. Repeat ten times.

Tips

1. I know there are a lot of details, but this exercise is the most important one you can do for aligning your body and finding and correcting the problem areas.

2. The pole must be *very* tight to get the alignment of the pelvic girdle. Once you gain control of your alignment, you can do the exercise without the pole.

3. If your knees do not face forward, but are hyperextended or turn-in, reread the discussion on The Knees at the opening of this chapter.

4. Make sure the can is at the back of the heel and not toward the arches. I do not want your ankles rolling in to hold onto the can. Review figures 1 and 4 for the correct way to balance.

Benefits

This exercise aligns and strengthens the feet, legs, and spine. The arches are stimulated and strengthened. It is one of the best preventions and cures for shin splints and flat feet.

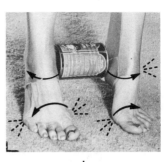

b

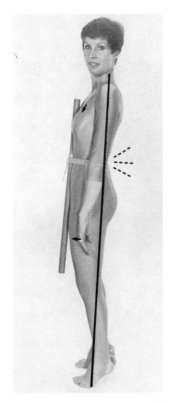

a   **Figure 3**
INCORRECT

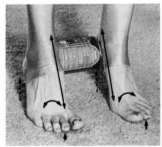

b

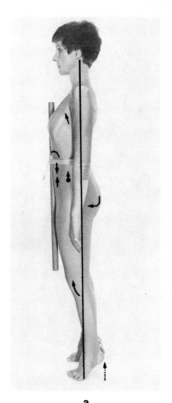

a

Figure 4

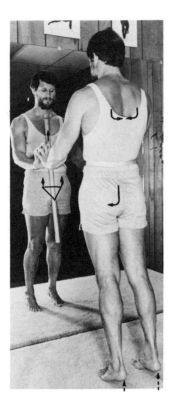

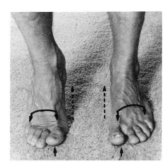

b

a

Figure 1

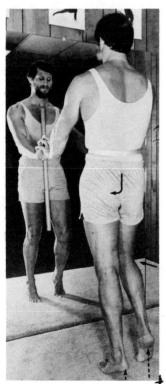

Figure 2

ACHILLES, ANKLE, AND CALF STRETCH AT MIRROR

Props

1. A 2½-foot pole or the attachment from a vacuum cleaner.
2. A belt with double-ring loops.
3. A full-length mirror, as in figure 1, or a small one that you can place on the floor.

Body Placement

1. Tie the pole *very* tightly around the waist.
2. Stand three feet away from the mirror.
3. Lean forward, placing only your fingertips on the mirror.

Technique

1. To get ready, inhale and elongate up the pole. While exhaling, contract your abdomen and rotate the pubic bone to the pole. Raise your toes and align your body.
2. Now, inhale and come up on the balanced balls of your feet, as in figure 1a. Look closely at figure 1b. Your feet should *not* roll in or out. Pretend you still have the can between your heels, as in the previous exercise.
3. While exhaling, bend the right knee to remain on the balls of your foot, as in figure 2. While you lower the left heel directly back, work hard to keep the toes of the left foot raised, as in figure 3a.
4. Repeat the Complete Breath as you work in this position. Watch to make sure you don't drop your arch. Don't lower the heel so far, if you have to roll the arch. See figure 3b.

5. Once you can lower an aligned foot with the toes extended, heels down, knees facing forward, and pubic bone on the pole, you can bend the elbows to create a blade squeeze and tilt the body forward to increase the stretch, as in figure 4.
6. Repeat, using the Complete Breath in this position to fine tune your alignment.
7. Raise your left foot to meet the right, as in figure 2.
8. Repeat the full sequence while lowering the right heel.
9. Repeat twice. It's how long you stay in the stretch that counts. Don't rush it.

Tips

1. Practice going up and down with your body at an angle and, at first, with the can between your heels to gain control in the alignment of the feet and back.
2. Do *not* lower your heels too low so you lose the alignment of the arch. If standing three feet from the mirror is too far for you, come in closer.
3. Once you have accomplished this exercise, you can do it without the mirror and pole. If you are outdoors, use a tree trunk or wall on a building for balance and support.
4. When standing three feet away gives you no stretch and when you have maintained your alignment in the neck, shoulder, hip, knee, and ankle, step back a little more.

Benefits

The ankles are stimulated and strengthened. This is good for flat feet. Also, the Achilles' tendons and calves are getting a good stretch. When doing this exercise correctly, the knees as well as the lower back are protected.

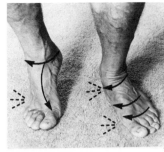

b
INCORRECT

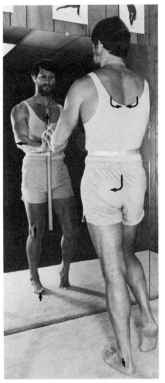

a

Figure 3

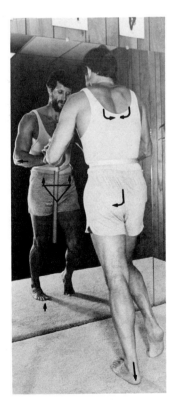

Figure 4

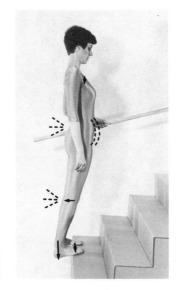

Figure 1

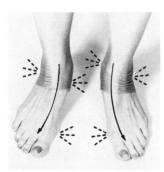

a   b

Figure 3
INCORRECT

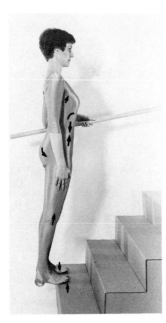

a

Figure 2
INCORRECT

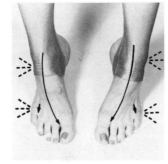

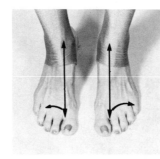

b

Figure 4

ACHILLES, ANKLE, AND CALF STRETCH AT STAIRS

Props

1. A stairway with a railing.
2. A can of food measuring 4½ inches tall.

Body Placement

1. Hold onto the railing.
2. Stand at the edge of the step and up on the balls of your feet with the can between your heels, as in figure 1.
3. Align your body as if you were wearing the pole, as in the previous exercises.

Technique

1. While inhaling, raise your toes and press the balls of the feet into the step. Now raise the heels and use the can to align the foot, as in figure 1.
2. Stay up there. Exhale and align the legs and upper body. Remember the position with the pole.
3. Inhale and elongate. While exhaling, contract your abdomen as you keep the body "toned" (in control). Lower the heels, as in figure 4a.
4. Hold for the count of four. Do *not* drop the heels, hyperextend the knees, or roll the ankles in or out, as in figures 2 and 3.
5. Look closely at figure 4. Throughout this exercise, keep a lifted arch, raised kneecap, tucked buttocks, and lifted chest.
6. Repeat six times.

Tips

1. After you can maintain the control and alignment, you may do the exercise without the can.
2. Do *not* grip with your toes. Keep them extended.
3. Remember to align the four front tires (balls of your feet).
4. If you are having difficulties with alignment, use the tied-pole technique.

Benefits

This exercise is extremely helpful for weak ankles. The Achilles' tendons and calves get a very good stretch, and the knees are protected.

BALANCE ON ONE LEG

Props

1. A chair.
2. A full-length mirror.

Body Placement

1. Stand with the chair at your side or at a mirrored wall, if possible.
2. Place your hand on the chair or wall for support.

Technique

1. Inhale, elongate the body, and bend the left knee. Draw the left foot up on the toes, as in figure 1.
2. Exhale and contract your abdomen while aligning the body. Bring the left ankle to the inside of the right knee, as in figure 2.
3. Inhale and maintain a lift in the body. Exhale and contract your abdomen. Align the body with the kneecaps lifted and facing forward. Keep your hips level, as in figure 4. Hold this position.
4. Do *not* let yourself slouch or lean into the hip, as in figures 3 a and b.
5. Repeat Technique step 3 for four breaths.
6. Come down and begin again with the other side.
7. Repeat two more times.

Variation

If you can sustain an aligned balance, take your hand off the chair or wall. Repeat Technique steps 1-6 without the chair or wall.

Tips

1. Tying the pole to you is most helpful in aligning and strengthening the body.
2. Don't be anxious to do it without support. When you do, you fall in the position of figures 3a and b.
3. Concentrate on the elongation upward and the balance on your four tires (balls of your feet).
4. It will help greatly if you fix your gaze on a spot on the floor about your height's distance away.

Benefits

This exercise builds confidence, strengthens the balance of your body, and energizes the feet.

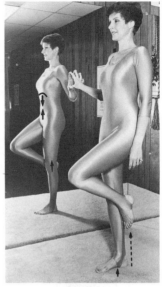
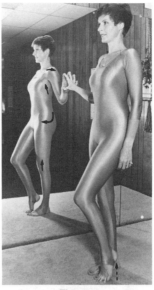

| Figure 1 | Figure 2 |

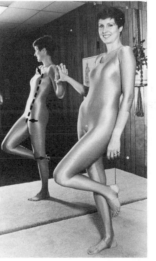

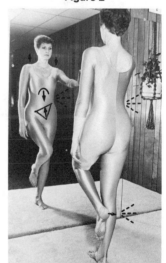

a   Figure 3   b

INCORRECT

Figure 4

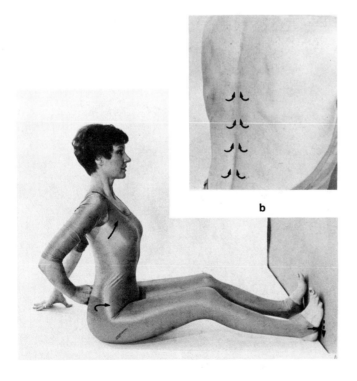

Figure 1
INCORRECT

b

TO ALIGN AND STRENGTHEN THE KNEE

Props

1. A wall or piece of furniture.

Body Placement

1. Place your feet up against wall, hip-width apart.
2. Do *not* sit slouched, as in figure 1.
3. Lean back, bend your knees, and arch the spine up into the body. Check with your hand, as in figure 2a. With your spine in, straighten the legs. You might have to move back to do so.

Technique

1. With both hands on the floor and the spine arched up into the body, inhale as you push the body upward.
2. Exhale and remain sitting straight up on the ischial bones, while you tighten the knees and draw them toward the thighs. Extend the heels to the wall. The legs and heels should be flat on the floor, with the heels pressed into the corner of the wall.
3. While inhaling, ease up on the kneecaps; but keep your body arched upward. Check to see that the spine is not protruding outward. Study figures 1b and 2b.
4. Exhale, tighten the whole leg, and work the back straighter and hands closer to the buttocks, as in figure 3. Looks easy, doesn't it!
5. Repeat Technique steps 3 and 4 four more times.

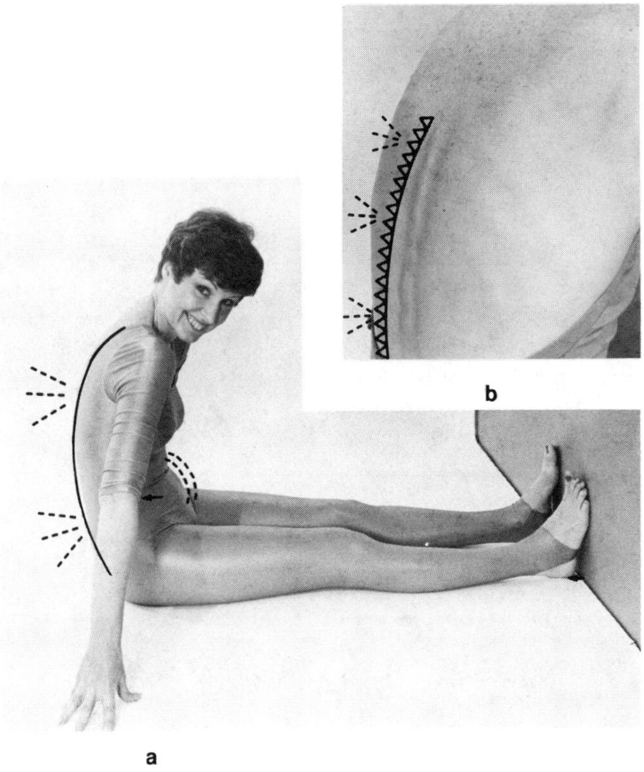

b

a

Figure 2

Variation

1. When going to the health club or therapy for your knee, make sure you apply the Technique steps, for the correct figure 4a.

2. Do *not* sit slackened, with your foot crooked, as in figure 4b. You are working the knee out of alignment because of poor foot and hip placement. The knee becomes strengthened in a twisted manner and can give you problems going up and down stairs in the future.

Tips

1. If it is hard on your hands to hold yourself up, place your elbows behind you on a low coffee table.

2. It's very important that you sit straight up on your ischial bones and that the spine is recessed, even if you have to sit leaning way back, more than in figure 2 with the legs straight.

3. Students with hyperextended knees *must* keep the heels on the floor. If they come up, place some weights on top of your feet.

4. This is a therapeutic exercise for those with hyperextended knees. Note how it makes the thighs work as they have never done so before. Don't worry about the action behind the knee—you are tightening weak ligaments.

Benefits

This exercise corrects the alignment of the knee joint and strengthens the whole leg and back.

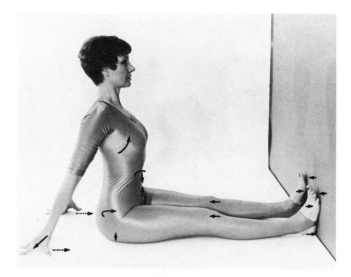

Figure 3

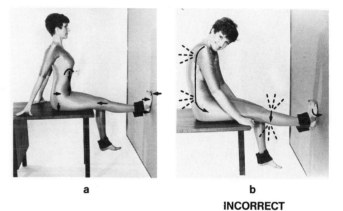

a

b

INCORRECT

Figure 4

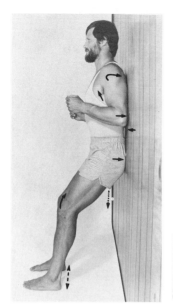

Figure 1

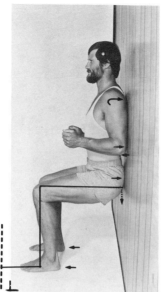

Figure 2

STRENGTHENER FOR HYPEREXTENDED KNEES— PHANTOM CHAIR

Props

1. A wall.

Body Placement

1. Lean your back against the wall and walk your feet out to where it's difficult to stand up, as in figure 1.
2. Place your upper arms, head, and sacrum against the wall. Lift your chest and create a blade squeeze.
3. Your *waist is off the wall*. Keep the natural lumbar curve.
4. Feet and knees are hip-distance apart.
5. Slide down the wall to form a right angle, as the lines indicate in figure 2. If your legs are like Dick's, look to the side. Adjust your feet and knees to a right angle. Keep them there. Come up, without moving your feet. Now, you are ready.

Technique

1. While inhaling, elongate the spine and raise the toes, as in figure 1.
2. Exhale and press your feet down, lifting the kneecaps toward the thighs. Keep pushing your feet so the sacrum is firm on the wall as you slide down, as in figure 2.
3. Come down to a controlled right angle. If you feel or look like figure 3, come up and repeat Body Placement steps 1-5.

4. When in a right angle, hold the position. Inhale and elongate. While exhaling, continue to push the feet down, without sliding. Count to ten. Come up while inhaling. I bet you're happy to be up!

5. Repeat five times. Work up to ten times, twice a day.

Tips

1. If one leg is stronger than the other, there is a tendency to slide down, tilting to one side. Have someone check you so you look as figure 4.

2. Keep the balance and work in the legs by continually pushing your feet down into the floor and by tightening the thighs toward the groin.

3. Once you have adjusted your feet to the right angle, put a strip of tape on the floor or rug (where the dotted line is in figure 2) to assure a right angle every time.

4. Remember to keep your waist off the wall without overarching it. Keep the natural lumbar curve.

5. Check your feet. Align your eight tires (balls and heels) with your toes up. Don't let your feet web out or roll in.

Benefits

Although valuable for anyone, this exercise, when done correctly, is especially good for those with hyperextended knees. It strengthens the feet, knees, and thighs and tightens the ligaments in the back of the knees.

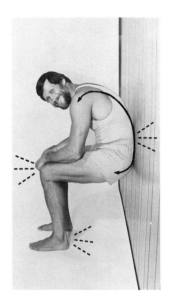

Figure 3
INCORRECT

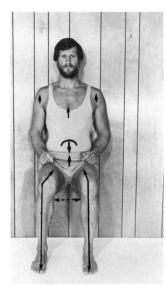

Figure 4

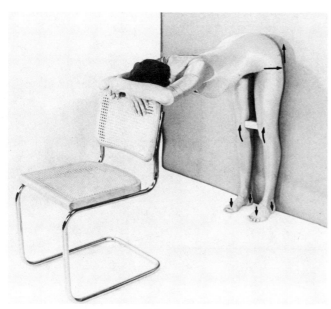

Figure 1

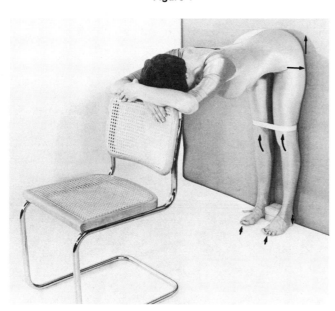

Figure 2

WORKING WITH PROBLEM KNEES

Props

1. For knock-knees and cross-eyed knees, use a block or can of food large enough to keep the legs and feet hip-width apart.
2. For bowed legs, use a belt.
3. For hyperextended knees, use a block or rolled towel.
4. Use a chair for balance.

Body Placement

1. Stand at the wall with your heels against the wall. Hold onto the chair for balance.

Technique

1. While inhaling, raise your toes. Lift the kneecaps toward your thighs and work the ischial bones up the wall.
2. While exhaling, extend the ischial bones and head in opposite directions, creating a blade squeeze and elongated spine.
3. Repeat steps 1 and 2 until you have worked your knees correctly, which means facing forward and straight.

Variation for Knock-Knees and Cross-eyed Knees

1. Place a block between your knees, as in figure 1.
2. Apply Technique steps 1-3, while you turn your knees to face forward with lifted kneecaps.
3. Align your feet into the floor. I know the feet want to turn out, but work the eight tires (balls and heels) down with lifted arches.

Variation for Bowed Legs

1. Tie a belt around the legs, just above the knees, and put a block of wood between the heels, as in figure 2.

2. With your feet hip-width apart, work them strongly into the floor.

3. Apply Technique steps 1-3, while you turn your knees to face forward, lifting the kneecaps.

4. Work your leg against the wall and away from the belt to bring them into an aligned position.

Variation for Hyperextended Knees

1. With your legs against the wall and your knees facing forward, keep your feet aligned and work them into the floor.

2. If you find you are still hyperextended (locking knees back) place a rolled towel, block, or book behind your knees, as in figure 3.

3. Really work the balls of the feet down. Strengthen the knees and thighs by raising them upward while keeping your heels down.

4. Apply Technique steps 1-3. I bet you never felt work like that in the legs before!

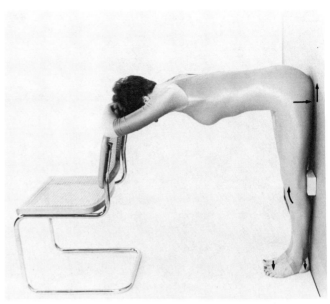

Figure 3

Tips

1. Doing these Variations will work the legs so the level of your back is aligned, but not tense. Use the chair for balance.

2. To check the alignment of your back, feel a smooth groove with the spine recessed into the body.

3. To strengthen the new alignment of the legs, it is important to work the feet down and the ischial bones up.

Benefits

These corrective exercises are most valuable for the named problems.

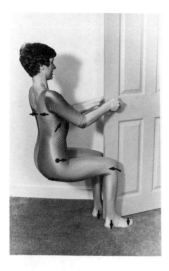

Figure 1

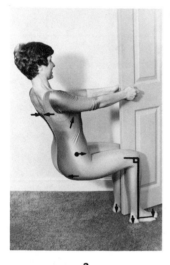

a

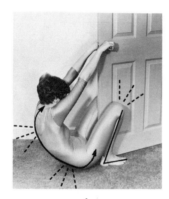

b

INCORRECT

Figure 2

SQUATTING KNEE STRENGTHENER

Props

1. A set of doorknobs in a door.

Body Placement

1. Hold onto the doorknobs with your feet parallel. The edge of the door lines up with the back of your heel, as in figure 1.
2. Lean back with straight arms, as if you are going to sit in a chair, as in figure 2a. Don't worry; you won't fall.
3. Throughout the Squatting exercise, the feet remain aligned with lifted arches.
4. Keep your knees over your ankles during the exercises, as in figures 1, 2, and 3.
5. At all times, the buttocks are arched backward and the spine is recessed, though not overarched.
6. Do *not* squat so low that you round your back and lose your balance, as in figure 2b.

Technique

1. While inhaling, push your feet down into the floor, extend your chest to the door, make a blade squeeze, and keep your arms straight.
2. Exhale and arch your buttocks back as if to sit in a chair. While keeping the blade squeeze, lower yourself to where you can maintain control and balance, as in figure 2.
3. Hold this position. Repeat steps 1 and 2 to work the feet stronger into the floor. This will align and strengthen the knees and back.
4. Do *not* drop down to where the knees are not over the ankles and where the back is rounded, as in figure 2b.
5. Come up by further pushing your feet down. Use your legs, not only your arms, to spring up.
6. Repeat four times.

Variation 1

1. Line your toes to the edge of the door, as in figure 3.
2. Repeat Technique steps 1-4, making sure your knees are over your ankles and your spine is recessed. You can check by holding on with one hand.
3. Repeat four times.

Variation 2

1. Assume a perfect posture position with your feet apart at hip-distance.
2. Inhale and raise your arms out front to shoulder level.
3. To lower, exhale and contract your abdomen. With the blades squeezing, keep your back straight and work, as in figure 4a. To come up, press your feet down with lifted arches and spring up from your legs.
4. If you went this far without raising your heels and you have kept the knees hip-width, with no knee pain, you are ready to go lower.
5. Repeat steps 1-3, leaning more forward and keeping a lift in the buttocks. Work lower, as in figure 4b.
6. Repeat four times *only* if you have no pain and if you can keep the heels down and the back flat. If so, good for you!

Tips

1. For students with bad knees, I have them start the exercise with their heels in line with the door. This takes most of the weight off the knees and still works them correctly.
2. If there is no pain, work your foot in small increments from the figure 1 position to the figure 3 position.
3. Throughout these exercises, the knees and thighs should be lifting upward toward the hip. This aligns the control of the kneecap.
4. Do *not* do these exercises if you have any sharp knee pain. It may be that you are not pressing and working your feet right or you may have a problem with your knees.
5. If your Archilles' tendons are short, it will be difficult for you to squat and keep your heels on the floor. Place a book under the heels. It should be thick enough so the heels can rest on it; but stretch is still felt in the Archilles' tendons.
6. Make sure you differentiate between sharp pain and the feeling that results from tired, hard-working legs. If done correctly, your legs should feel good and springy when walking.
7. Another caution: Be careful *not* to overarch the lower back ("rut feeling"). Balance the pelvis.

Benefits

This exercise strengthens the knees, legs, and ankles. It develops the thigh muscles and corrects minor leg problems.

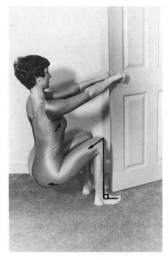

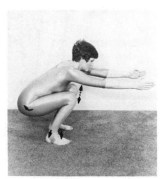

Figure 3

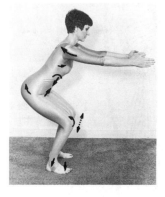

a

b

Figure 4

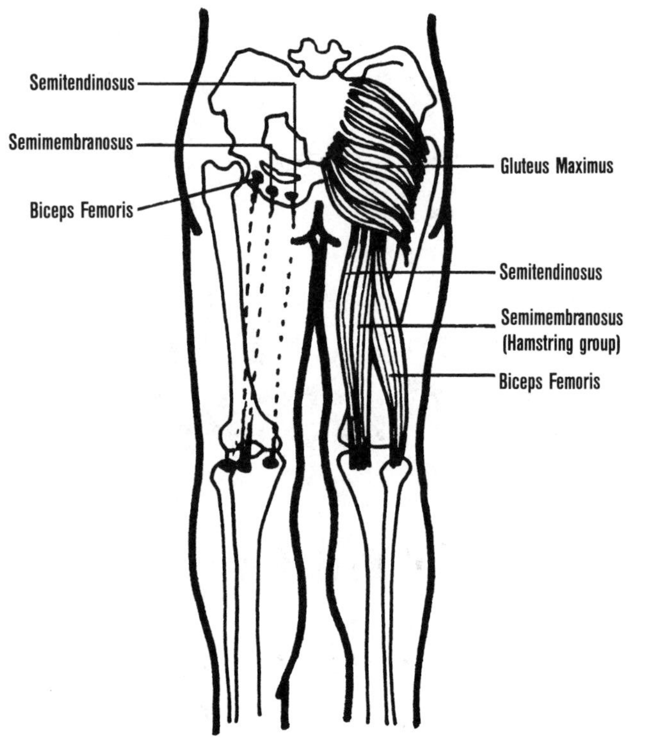

2. Hamstrings, Thighs, Buttocks, and Groin

Figure 1

Semitendinosus

Semimembranosus

Biceps Femoris

Gluteus Maximus

Semitendinosus

Semimembranosus (Hamstring group)

Biceps Femoris

"That's life," you say, "I can't do anything about my tight hamstrings and groin and big butt—I've had a big butt all my life." I hear this all the time, but I say that you *can* change them and that you alone *can* do something. It's never too late to free yourself from the programming of your past, to assume responsibility for your body, and to discover possibilities you don't even suspect.

In this chapter and throughout the book, I will show you ways of investigating the natural methods of working the body as an indissoluble whole—ways that will help you shape your body. The goal is not to have you escape from your body, but to avoid having your body continue to escape you through pain and limited activity.

You can unlearn the bad habits that make you favor certain parts of the body, causing overdevelopment and deformity, and neglect others. Reconsider the unintelligent automatic movements of your body, leave some off, reconstruct others, and add new ones to discover the body's efficiency and spontaneity.

If I speak to you with so much conviction and enthusiasm, it's because I see these battles won every day!

Hamstrings, Thighs, and Buttocks

One of the most misunderstood exercises is the hamstring stretching routine. No football or track season goes by without numerous reports of pulled hamstrings and/or thigh muscles. The majority of these muscle tears result from improper or imbalanced strengthening of the thigh muscles.

To stretch the hamstrings properly requires a knowledge of how they work and what effects they have on other parts of the body. The hamstrings attach to two joints: the pelvis and the knees; therefore, the health of the hamstrings influences both of these joints. Proper stretching of the hamstrings can increase the fluidity in the knees and back, thereby relieving many complaints. If the hamstrings are too tight, they literally pull the pelvis down and can cause misalignment in the back, hips, or knees. It is imperative to stretch the hamstrings not only completely, but also correctly.

The hamstrings consist of three long, strong muscles on the back of each thigh that attach to the ischial bones, as in figure 1. From this attachment the three muscles cross the hip socket, traverse down the back of the thigh, cross the knee joint, and insert into the lower leg bones below the knee. Because of these "ties," the hamstrings influence and/or move the lower back, hip sockets, and knees.

Every day I see people with pulled groins and/or hamstrings because they are stretching incorrectly. For instance, when they bend over to touch their toes (There is no great virtue in touching toes; it gets a lot of people into trouble.), they do so by rounding the back, bending forward from the waist with the buttocks tucked down, and positioning the knees in any direction, as in figure 2. This means most of the movement and stretching is coming from the back, which creates back strain. The knees are either hyperextended or turned inward, which weakens them. The people think they are stretching their hamstrings; but, before the hams ever get a decent stretch, they have done damage to their back or knees.

Always align your posture first. Then continually check yourself. See if your feet are parallel and your knees straight forward and lifted. (See section III, chapter 2.) Keep your back straight. When you move, move the entire torso forward by lifting the buttocks up and extending the ribs outward and forward. The rotation comes from the hips, not from a strained back. See figure 3 for the correct position.

The first exercise, Hamstring Stretch at Wall, ensures an aligned back on the floor. The natural lumbar curve is monitored by the pole so that the stretch comes from the entire leg and heel. For some of you, it will be difficult to straighten the leg out. Be patient. You are feeling all you can take in the leg at this time, even if the leg is bent. Make sure the pole is comfortable. Remember, it's not how far you can go that counts; it's how *correct* you are in your method of getting there.

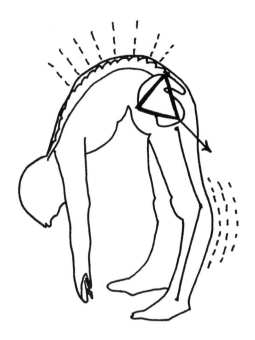

Figure 2
INCORRECT

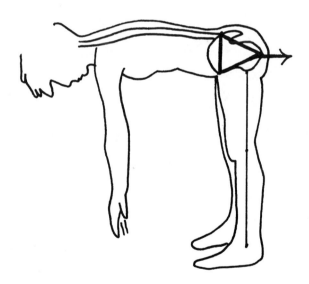

Figure 3

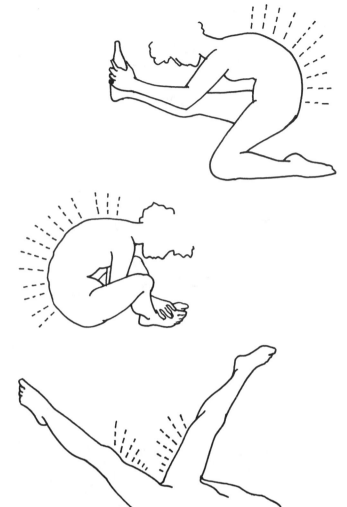

Figure 4

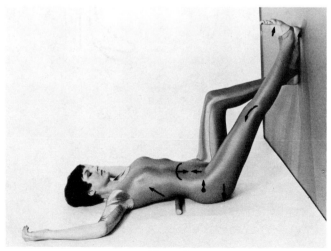

Figure 1

Groin

When people come to me with a pulled groin, I ask them to show me the stretches they are doing. The most popular ones appear in figure 4. When they show me their exercises, their pain becomes sharper. They then tell me they have a high tolerance for pain, thinking that the pain is good for them. The statement "no pain, no gain" is what got them into trouble in the first place. Their hips and lower backs are not aligned, thus they put a tremendous strain on the sciatic nerve and lower back and rip the groin.

I have written the Answer to Hurdler's Stretch in this chapter for those of you blessed with flexible hips so you will know the *right* execution of the exercise and save yourself from eventual injury. Unless you can sit with both ischial bones even and the spine recessed, I recommend that *no* one do the standard Hurdler's Stretch because of the way it is practiced. I believe it is high on the list of the most dangerous exercises—along with Toe-Touching and Sit-Ups. The standard Hurdler's Stretch can gradually cause harmful stretching of the ligament on the inside of the knee and enormous stress in the meniscus cartilage in the knee. It stretches the muscles and ligaments in the groin region farther than they were intended to go, not to mention what it does to the back and hips.

Tight hamstrings and groin muscles are also detrimental to proper alignment. They can change the four natural curves of the spine by exaggerating them and making the back muscles compensate for the new alignment, as shown in figure 4. The overall effect is one of compression and strain, resulting in possible back and groin misery. Remember, these pitfalls *can* be avoided with correct stretching of the hamstrings and groin.

HAMSTRING STRETCH AT WALL

Props

1. A wall.
2. Two long neckties tied together at the wide end, measuring approximately eight feet long.
3. A one-inch thick by twelve-inch long pole or a magazine rolled up to measure one inch in diameter, held together with rubber bands.

Body Placement

1. Lie down, with both feet on the wall. Bend the left knee to form a right angle, as in figure 1.
2. Balance on your sacrum. The pole should be comfortable under your waist.
3. Your chest is lifted up and the shoulder blades are flat. If needed, use your elbows to align your upper body.

Technique

1. While inhaling, elongate the spine. Exhale and slide your right heel up the wall. With your toes toward your face, lift the kneecap toward the thigh, as in figure 1.
2. Hold the position and use a Complete Breath. Make sure your spine is not pressing into the pole and you are anchored on the tailbone edge of the sacrum.
3. On the third exhale, contract your abdomen and balance on the sacrum. Lift the right leg one inch off the wall. Hold for five counts.
4. Return the heels and repeat with the left leg.
5. Repeat the cycle three more times.

Variation 1

1. Place the wide part of the tie against the ball of the foot. With your elbows on the floor, grip the tie taut, as in figure 2.
2. Inhale and elongate the spine off the pole, anchoring on the sacrum.
3. While exhaling, contract your abdomen and tighten the leg straight, (not locked back).
4. Inhale again. Without pulling the leg with the tie, exhale and use your abdominals to advance the legs forward.
5. Now, hold the leg there with the tie and use it as leverage to inhale and elongate off the pole.
6. Repeat steps 2-5, until the leg is free to balance, as in figure 3. Take the pole away and advance it even further.
7. Hold the leg at each stage for the count of five.
8. Make sure you dip the tailbone downward.
9. Return the leg to the right-angle position.
10. Repeat with the other leg.

Variation 2

1. Slide out so the left heel is where the floor and wall meet, as in figure 4.
2. Place the ties across the ball of the right foot and hold them with your left hand, keeping the arm straight.
3. Place the right thumb where the thigh and hip meet. Rotate the muscle to the side and push it away. This aids in aligning the pelvic triangle. Work the ischial bones toward each other, as in figure 4.
4. Repeat steps 2-10 in Variation 1.

Tips

1. Do *not* go on to the Variations unless your legs can be extended completely straight.
2. If you can't straighten your legs, take about five breaths and keep working; but don't force yourself. Breathe into it.
3. If your legs are tight, there is a tendency to roll up your buttocks and press the spine into the pole. Do *not* do that.

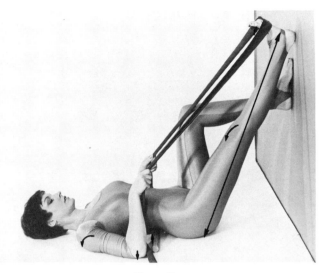

Figure 2

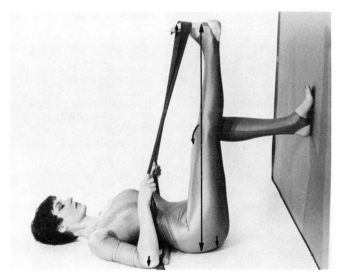

Figure 3

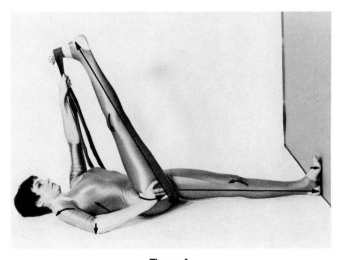

Figure 4

4. Keep the spine off the pole and the tailbone end of the sacrum anchored to floor. Don't worry, the leg will get straight . . . it's your tight hamstrings that hinder you.
5. As you advance your raised leg forward, make sure you don't roll your thighs out to the side. Keep your hips even and level as a horizontal pelvic triangle. It helps to keep the inner thighs toward each other.

Benefits

This exercise works to align and free the hips, stretches the hamstrings, tones the abdomen, and strengthens the legs.

HUGGING HAMSTRING STRETCH

Props

1. A wall.

Body Placement

1. Place the heels two feet away from the wall.
2. Bend over to hug the legs, as in figure 1. Draw the ribs against the thighs and raise your toes.

Technique

1. Inhale and elongate the ribs down the thighs.
2. While exhaling, push the feet into the floor as you slide your buttocks up the wall, as in figure 2.
3. Hold for the count of six. Then ease the legs a little.
4. Repeat steps 1-3 five times.

Variation 1

1. To aid the buttocks in the lift, take your fingers and give a push upward to the ischial bones, as in figure 3.
2. Repeat Technique steps 1-4. Relax.

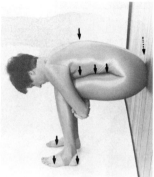
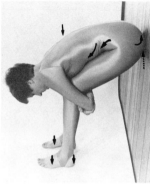

Figure 1   **Figure 2**

Variation 2

1. Keeping the ribs on the thighs, spread your fingers to the wall, and make a blade squeeze, as in figure 4.   .
2. Inhale and elongate the spine.
3. While exhaling, feed the spine deep into the body as you continue to push the feet. How's that for a good stretch?
4. Repeat Technique steps 1-4. Relax.

Tips

1. The object is to straighten your legs. If it's not an effort to do so, place your feet closer to the wall so it will be more difficult to do. This stretches the hamstrings without the temptation of locking your knees back.
2. Remember, it's how well you're working or feeling it and how well you're getting there that counts, not how far you get.
3. If you open the space between your ribs and thighs too much, you lose the stretch in the hamstrings.
4. You must keep pushing down with the feet to go up with the ischial bones.

Benefits

This is an excellent hamstring exercise for those with hyper-extended knees. It protects the knees and strengthens the legs.

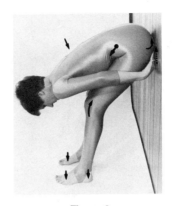

Figure 3

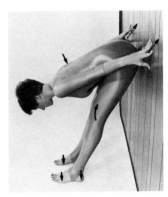

Figure 4

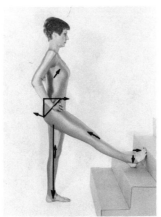

Figure 1

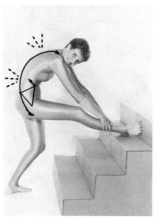

Figure 2
INCORRECT

STANDING HAMSTRING STRETCH

Props

1. A set of stairs with walls on each side.

Body Placement

1. Stand facing the stairs with the right leg on the second step, as in figure 1.
2. Do *not* go higher on the step if you look like figure 2 (even if you have gone higher with a rounded back). This method requires aligning the hips, which makes a big difference.
3. With your hands on the walls, move the left foot so it is straight under the body and place the right foot up against the upper step, as in figure 1.
4. With your hands on your hips, align your hips so the pubic bone and frontal hipbones are exactly vertical and the crest of the hipbones are level.
5. You may have to bend the right leg to bring the pelvic triangle in line.
6. To hold this alignment in place, keep your ischial bones moving toward each other. Don't open your hip out to the side.

Technique

1. Inhale and elongate the ribs out of the waist, while standing very firm on the left leg. Place your right thumb on the thigh just under the hipbone.
2. While exhaling, rotate that tight muscle to the side and down, moving your ischial bones toward each other. Hold this position.
3. Now that you have aligned your hips, take your right hand and feel to be sure your spine is recessed. If it's not, don't bend forward until you work it in.
4. Inhale and place your hand back on the thigh muscle to give you leverage to elongate and lift the chest up and forward.

5. Exhale. While squeezing the ischial bones toward each other, aim them back and upward. Draw your hipbones forward from the pubic bone, as in figure 3.
6. Hold for five counts and continue working steps 4 and 5 for six Complete Breaths. Work your spine forward, as in figures 4a and b.
7. Lower your leg and repeat with the left leg.

Variation

1. If you can execute this exercise completely and have no stretch in the right leg, place it on the next step; but do not go higher than your hip.
2. Apply Technique steps 1-7 with your leg at the new level. Do *not* round your back. Keep the spine recessed, as in figure 4.

Tips

1. When the hips and back are checked and aligned, it is helpful to use the wall for balance and lift.
2. Make sure you pay attention to aligning the leg on the floor; but do not hyperextend. It works an important action in the hips.
3. To review: Alignment of the standing leg means the toes are raised and the knee is eased (not locked) and lifted upward. Ground the four tires of the foot with lifted arches into the floor.
4. Don't force this exercise. For some, just standing straight with the foot on the second step will be beneficial.
5. Remember, I *don't* believe in no pain, no gain. You should be aware of the proper muscles you are working and breathe into them.

Benefits

This exercise is excellent for aligning and strengthening the standing leg. It also aligns and works the hips and lower back. For a bonus, the hamstrings are stretched.

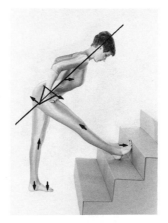

Figure 3

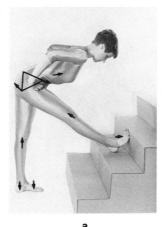

a

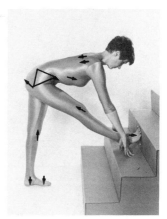

b

Figure 4

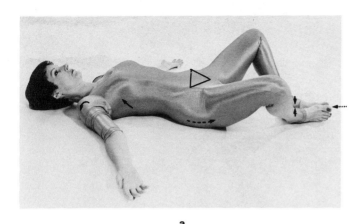

a

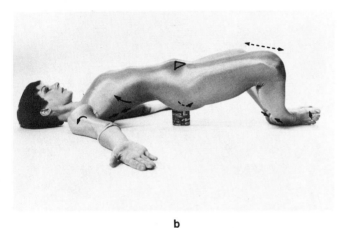

b

Figure 1

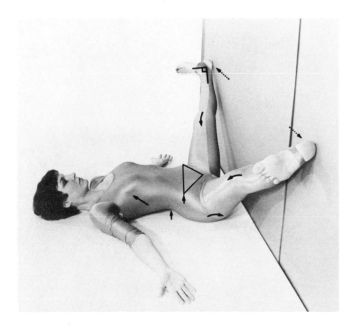

Figure 2

GROIN STRETCH

Props

1. Two blocks or tuna cans covered with a folded facecloth for comfort.
2. A wall.
3. A one-inch thick pole or rolled-up magazine.
4. A tie or belt.

Body Placement

1. Lie down, with your buttocks tucked downward and the pelvic triangle level. Your chest is open and rests on flat shoulder blades

Technique

1. For the Frog Leg Spread, draw your heels toward your groin with the soles of the feet together.
2. If your knees are higher than your hipbones, as in figure 1a, place one or two cans under your sacrum to help open and relax the groin, as in figure 1b.
3. Make sure you don't feel any jamming in the lower back. If so, you need to align your pelvic triangle and lengthen the spine.
4. Inhale as you elongate. While exhaling, contract the abdomen and let the legs relax their way down toward the floor.
5. Continue step 4 for ten Complete Breaths. Draw the legs in and together to relax. Don't worry, they'll come back together!

Variation 1, figure 2, Spread Eagle

1. Slide your buttocks to the wall. Dip your tailbone downward so the pole can fit through. Once you maintain the one-inch space, you don't need the pole.
2. If the pole doesn't fit, slide away from the wall until it does fit and the pelvic triangle is level.
3. Repeat Technique steps 3-5 with your legs open wide. Extend the heels with the knees raised toward the thighs, as in figure 2. Keep your knees in line with the hips and feet. Don't roll them toward the floor.

Variation 2, figure 3, Split Sacrum Balance

1. Bend your knees to line up over the hip bones and extend your heels, as in figure 3.
2. Balance on your sacrum with the pole being comfortable. Place a hand on the inside of the thighs.
3. Inhale and elongate the spine. While exhaling, maintain the pelvic triangle and let your legs lower on their own, as in figure 3.

4. Inhale and lift the chest, making a blade squeeze. While exhaling, dip to the tailbone and contract your abdomen, as you apply a little pressure with your hands.

5. Repeat steps 3 and 4 for six breaths. Do *not* push hard on your legs. Feel them lower on their own under your hands.

6. Draw your legs up and in and give them a good hug. Tell them they did a good job!

Variation 3, figure 4, Spinal Squeeze

1. Lower your feet to the floor, keep the knees bent, and draw up the left knee. Place interlaced fingers just below the bottom of the knee, as in figure 4. If you can't reach a good grip, place a tie or belt across the shin and hold on at the sides.

2. Anchoring on your sacrum, inhale a deep breath and lift your chest and ribs toward the knee.

3. Keep your shoulders and head on the floor. Do *not* roll up into a ball, as in figure 4a.

4. Exhale. *Don't* bring your knee to your chest. Use the knee as leverage to lift the ribs and chest. Squeeze the spine up into body. Hold for a count of six.

5. Keep the waist off the floor by dipping the tailbone down.

6. Ease the grip on the knee for each inhale. Repeat steps 2 and 4 two more times. Straighten out the right leg and extend the heels, while pushing the leg into floor. Hold for a count of six. Then stretch the left leg out and lower.

7. Repeat step 6, but bend the right knee.

8. Repeat the cycle three more times.

Tips

1. Because the curl-up position is practiced widely, study the differences in figure 4a and b and review the Technique. For the most beneficial effect, it's important you do it right. The curl-up position protrudes the tummy; rounds the back and shoulders; and presses the back out and into the floor, which doesn't give it protection.

2. The psoas muscle comes from the lower back and into the groin. When you hear of a pulled groin, it could be the psoas. When the pelvic triangle is not aligned, as it is not in most standard exercises, any movement can cause physical aggravation. So pay close attention to the directions.

3. If you started in the Frog Leg Spread with two cans, check periodically that your knees are level with your hips. If so, use one can or none at all.

Benefits

This is a very therapeutic exercise for the groin area and inner-thigh region. It also helps to adjust the hips.

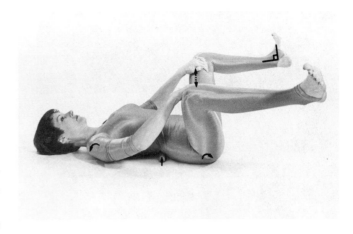

Figure 3

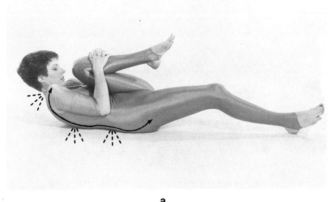

a
INCORRECT

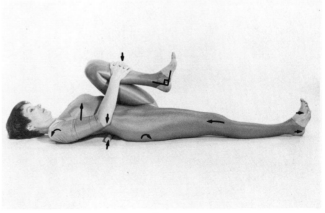

b

Figure 4

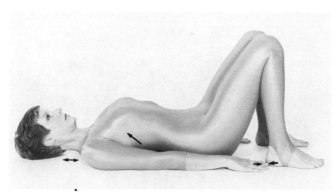

Figure 1

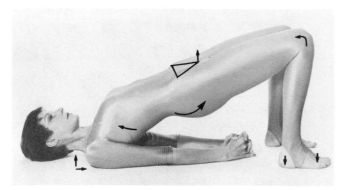

Figure 2

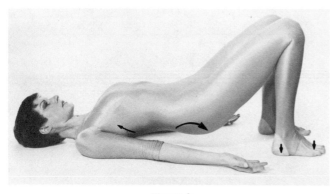

Figure 3

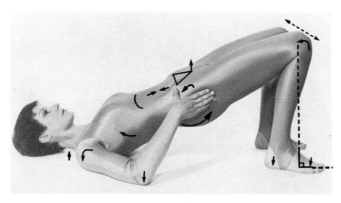

Figure 4

BURNING BUTT

Props

None

Body Placement

1. Lie down and bend your knees. Keep the feet a little wider than hip-distance apart so the heels come to the tips of your fingers.
2. Adjust your head so your neck is elongated, as in figure 1.

Technique

1. Inhale and press your feet into the floor—all eight tires worth! While exhaling, roll the buttocks up, leading with the rotated action of the tailbone.
2. Inhale with your arms straight on the floor. Clasp your hands beneath you and squeeze your shoulder blades together, while walking your shoulders in together and away from your neck. Your cervical spine should be lifted completely from the floor, as in figure 2.
3. While exhaling, keep your chest up and lower your hips, as if to sit down, as in figure 3.
4. Inhale and extend the sternum. As you exhale, contract the abdominals and rib cage, while the frontal hipbones and floating ribs draw toward each other. Put your hands on the hipbones, as in figure 4.
5. Inhale into the back of the ribs. While exhaling, contract the abdomen and rotate the pelvis by scooping up the tailbone. This enables you to squeeze the pubic bone higher than your hipbones. Your fingers are pulling your hips toward your waist and downward, as in figure 4.
6. Repeat step 5 three more times to increase your rotation.
7. Come down and rest.
8. Repeat the exercise three more times, taking seven breaths. Now, you know why it's called the Burning Butt!

Tips

1. Make sure your cervical spine is off the floor, so you can squeeze your arms and blades together.
2. Keep your ankles in line with your knees, forming a right angle, as the dotted line in figure 4 shows. It is very common to be in too close, as I am. This can aggravate the knee. So check your alignment.
3. If you tend to open your knees wider than your ankles, put a belt around your thighs to keep the correct distance.
4. This is not an arched back, but an inclined spine. Feel with your fingers that you maintain a smooth groove.

Benefits

This exercise works off fatty deposits and firms the legs, thighs, hips, and abdomen. It also loosens the neck and shoulder region.

KNEELING THIGH TILT

Props

1. A 2½-foot pole or the attachment from a vacuum.
2. A nylon belt with two rings to slide closed.

Body Placement

1. Tie the pole on you *very* tightly.
2. Kneel with your knees and feet hip-distance apart.
3. Place your hands on the front of the thighs, tuck in your chin, and shrug the shoulders forward.
4. Keep your knees hip-distance apart; but squeeze the knees inward in their skin to bring them up on top of kneecaps, as in figure 1.

Technique

1. Inhale and elongate the sternum up the pole. While exhaling, contract your abdomen and rotate the hips by tucking in your tailbone to push the pubic bone to the pole, as in figure 2.
2. While inhaling, keep the pubic bone and sternum on the pole. Exhale slowly and tilt your body in a straight line, as in figure 3. Hold for a count of six. Come up on your inhale. Good sport!
3. As you are in the tilt and holding the position, continue rotating the pubic bone to the pole and squeezing the knees.
4. Repeat steps 1-3 five more times.

Variation

1. You are ready for the variation only when you can tilt with control and not feel it in the knees or lower back.
2. Raise your arms and bend at the elbow, as in figure 4.
3. Repeat steps 1-4 without moving the pubic bone or sternum away from the pole.

Tips

1. The clue in this tilt is to keep the knees squeezing inward. This tightens the buttocks and helps to maintain the continual rotation in the hips.
2. Don't let your head arch back. Keep the chin tucked in.
3. When you feel you have gained the control of a straight spine, you may do this tilt without using the pole.

Benefits

This exercise is an excellent stretch for the thighs. It strengthens the knees and back and makes the feet more flexible.

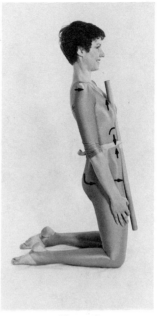

Figure 1

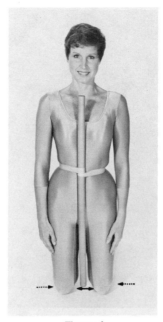

Figure 2

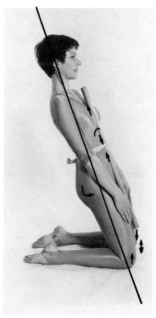

Figure 3

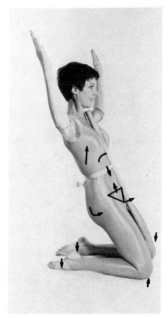

Figure 4

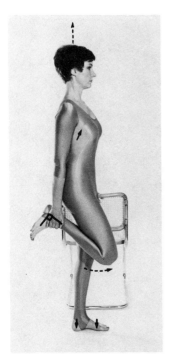

a

Figure 1

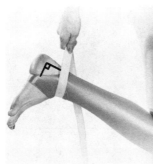

b

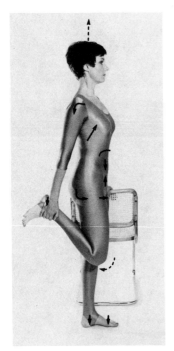

Figure 2

QUADRICEPS STRETCH

Props

1. A chair.
2. Optional, a double-looped belt.

Body Placement

1. Holding onto a chair, stand on your left leg as you bend the right knee and grasp the ankle (not the arch) with the right hand.
2. Bring the knee forward, as in figure 1a.

Technique

1. Move the right knee forward and stand up straight in perfect posture. Secure the left foot and leg by aligning them. Don't hang onto the chair.
2. Inhale and elongate. While exhaling, contract the abdomen and tuck by rotating the tailbone. This will bring the pubic bone forward and in alignment with the hipbones. You need a vertical pelvic triangle.
3. Inhale and elongate. While exhaling, shrug your shoulders back and create a blade squeeze. Maintain a tightly aligned pelvic girdle.
4. Continue to tighten the rotation as you draw the right thigh in line with the left thigh, as in figure 2.
5. Continue the Breathing Rhythm, as you repeat steps 2-4. The right leg pulls the right arm taut. There is a downward and upward pull. Keep the pubic bone rotating forward, as in figure 3.

6. As you gain stretch in the thigh, control of the pelvis, and balance, let go of the chair, as in figure 4.
7. In this position, the balance is maintained by the continued pulling and arching of the right leg, giving a bow-like action.
8. There is more action and leverage behind you, even though you are reaching forward.
9. Hold this balance as long as you can and come out as slowly as you went into it. Good for you! Rest and repeat with the left leg.

Tips

1. It is important that you keep a tight rotation in the pelvis. Do not just open the hip out to the side and pull the leg up.
2. Remember, it is how correctly you are working an area that counts, not how far up you get—at the mercy of a bad hip or pulled groin.
3. Most of you are getting all the stretch you can handle right now, as in figure 2. That's fine! In time the *body will tell* you when it is ready for more.
4. Tying a pole to yourself is very helpful in monitoring the pubic bone to keep the pelvic triangle in line.
5. If it is difficult to grab onto the ankle and work the hip correctly, a looped belt will work fine, as in figure 1b.
6. It is very helpful to fix your gaze on a spot on the floor, about your height's distance away.

Benefits

This exercise develops coordination and balance. It also stretches the thighs and shoulders and strengthens the hips.

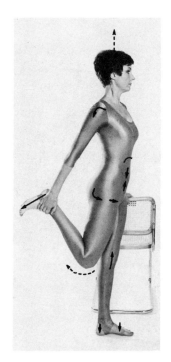

Figure 3

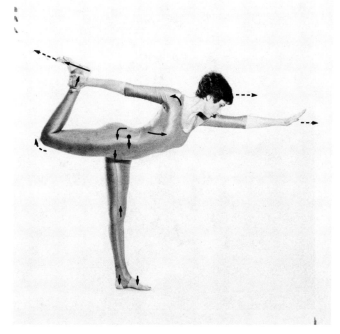

Figure 4

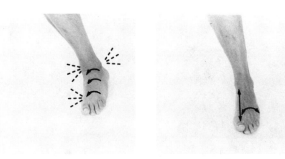

a b

INCORRECT

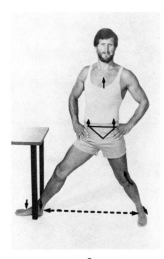

c

Figure 1

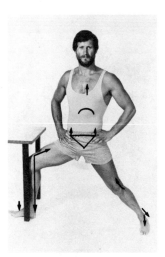

Figure 2

FRONT FACING PLUNGE

Props

1. A corner of a doorway or furniture.

Body Placement

1. Stand with your feet four feet apart. Place the right ankle at the corner, as in figure 1c.
2. Pivot on the heel, turning the right foot out and the left foot in.
3. The right knee should be in line with the right foot. So, if needed, turn your knee and let your left hip cooperate in the alignment. The right heel is in line with the arch of the left foot.
4. Your left foot should be planted firmly on the floor, as in figure 1b, not as in figure 1a. The knee should be lifted and aligned with the foot.
5. The pelvic triangle should face forward and be vertical. Don't force it forward at the sacrifice of the knees, which will turn you out of alignment.
6. As you lower, your spine takes the action of a straight plumb line.

Technique

1. Inhale and press your feet (the eight tires) firmly into the floor. Raise your kneecaps and lift your trunk up, while keeping your shoulders down.
2. While exhaling, contract your abdomen and tuck the tailbone to bring the pubic bone forward. Maintain the pelvic triangle, as in figure 1c.
3. Inhale and sustain the lift. While exhaling, keep the right foot and knee firm. Bend the knee to the side of the corner, as in figure 2.
4. Repeat steps 1-3 as you work yourself down to a right angle, with the spine like a plumb line, as in figure 4.

5. Do *not* lose the alignment of the feet and knees and control of the pelvic triangle to achieve the right angle, as in figure 3. What counts is that you are working your groin and gaining stamina in the legs. Remember, the priority of purposes are alignment and balance.

6. Use five breaths and work into your right-angle position. Come out and repeat with the left leg. Repeat the cycle two more times.

Breathing Rhythm

1. Inhale means to elongate and reinforce body balance by grounding your position.

2. Exhale means to contract the abdomen, secure a vertical pelvic triangle, and then work into the positon only if the body is open and accepts the advancement.

3. Hold means to hold out the exhalation for a pause and hold the balance of the position so the muscles can adjust in their stretch. What a stretch, huh?

4. Repeat the cycle.

5. When you have had enough, come out of it and repeat with the other side.

Tips

1. It is very helpful to do this in front of a mirror, facing sideways and toward the front. Use a chair for your knee and support.

2. It helps to stroke the thighs with your hands, as the arrows show.

3. Look closely at figures 1a and b. Don't forget to be attentive to the correct support in the left foot. You keep a lifted arch, but keep pressure under the ball of the big toe.

4. It is of great importance to feel very grounded in this exercise. Once you can accomplish keeping the right knee over the ankle, you can work without the table.

Benefits

This exercise strengthens the feet, ankles, knees, thighs, and hips, while also stretching the groin and thighs.

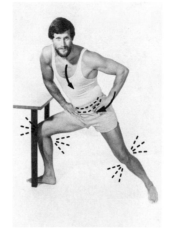 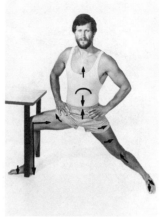

Figure 3
INCORRECT

Figure 4

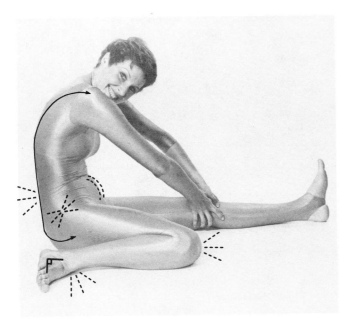

Figure 1
INCORRECT

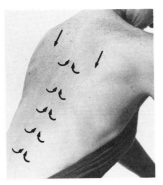

Figure 2

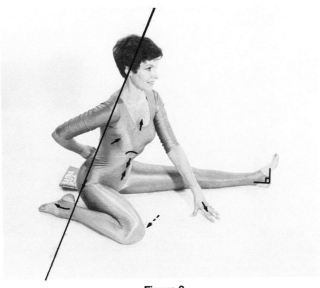

Figure 3

ANSWER TO HURDLER'S STRETCH

I have chosen not to teach the classic Hurdler's Stretch, as in figure 1, because of the way I see it done. Although it can be done correctly, I usually see results that show disrespect for and harm to the body. The hips are being strained when only one side of the buttocks is on the floor. With the back rounded, a tremendous strain and pull is put on the back. Also, the groin is being aggravated by the uneven hip—need I say more?

Props

1. A folded blanket or stack of books.

Body Placement

1. Sit on the floor with your left leg out to the side. Your right leg is bent with the foot toward the buttocks. Open the knees out to the side.
2. Sit up in a straight position. The spine should be centered between the legs. Make sure both of your ischial bones are grounded to the floor.
3. To free the hips to work right, arch the back, as in figure 2, by leaning on your arms and pressing those ischial bones into the floor. Feel for the smooth groove, as in figure 3.
4. Inhale and continue repeating steps 2 and 3. Elongate your recessed spine forward toward the floor in front of you.
5. Don't force to get down. It's the stretch in the thighs you want, and for most of you just working, as in figure 2, is all you can take. That's fine!

Breathing Rhythm

1. Inhale means to elongate and, at the same time, anchor your foundation on the two ischial bones.
2. Exhale means you secure your alignment and a firm foundation. Do *not* pull yourself forward, letting your ischial bones lift off the floor.
3. Hold means to hold the breath out for six counts and work to advance into the position. When the body opens to it, draw your attention within.
4. The action of the hips is like a ratchet wrench.

5. With the spine recessed, take your hand and make sure there is a smooth groove. If you feel a bumpy spine, sit up on a folded blanket or on books, the height of which depends on what you need to work your spine in and sit straight up on both of those ischial bones. Do *not* sit as in figures 4 and 5.

Technique

1. While inhaling, elongate your spine. Use your fingers for an aid in the lift and also to arch your lower back so that the ischial bones are grounded straight down (as the base for this exercise).
2. With your thighs spread wide apart, exhale and extend the left heel. With your toes toward your face, raise the kneecap and press the leg down as well as extend it. The right leg is bent wide to the side and pressed down.
3. Inhale and elongate. At the same time, ground your ischial bones. Exhale and, with the ischial bones down, extend the spine forward. Keep the body centered between the legs, as in figure 6.
4. Use five breaths, while elongating and stretching. Come out slowly and reverse positions. Repeat the cycle two more times.

Tips

1. As you advance, check periodically to make sure your spine is still recessed. Otherwise, your hips will lock backward, as in figure 5.
2. If your spine really sticks out when you sit on the floor, sit on the stack of books piled up to five inches high and work down from there. It would be beneficial to study the exercise called Sitting Up on the Ischial Bones in the next chapter.
3. Do not advance forward, as in figure 6, with more than a one-inch book. Stay up, as in figure 3 and work the rotation of the hips until you are on the book or until you no longer need it. Your hips are now open enough to go to the next step and advance (ratchet wrench) forward.

Benefits

When executed in this fashion, this exercise is an excellent stretch for the thighs and groin. It aligns the hips and makes them more flexible.

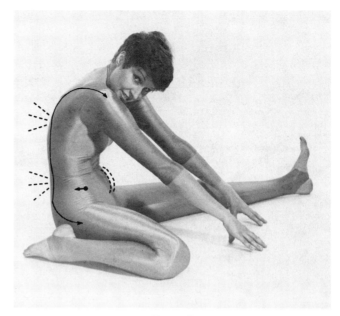

Figure 4
INCORRECT

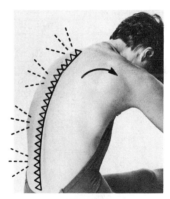

Figure 5
INCORRECT

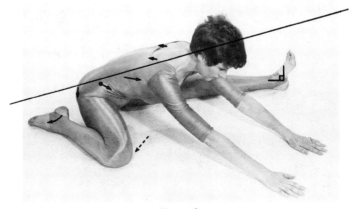

Figure 6

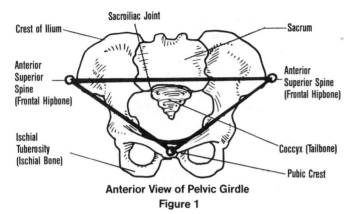

**Anterior View of Pelvic Girdle
Figure 1**

Crest of Ilium
Sacroiliac Joint
Sacrum
Anterior Superior Spine (Frontal Hipbone)
Anterior Superior Spine (Frontal Hipbone)
Ischial Tuberosity (Ischial Bone)
Coccyx (Tailbone)
Pubic Crest

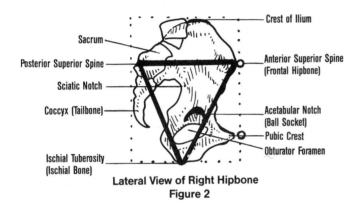

**Lateral View of Right Hipbone
Figure 2**

Sacrum
Crest of Ilium
Posterior Superior Spine
Anterior Superior Spine (Frontal Hipbone)
Sciatic Notch
Coccyx (Tailbone)
Acetabular Notch (Ball Socket)
Pubic Crest
Obturator Foramen
Ischial Tuberosity (Ischial Bone)

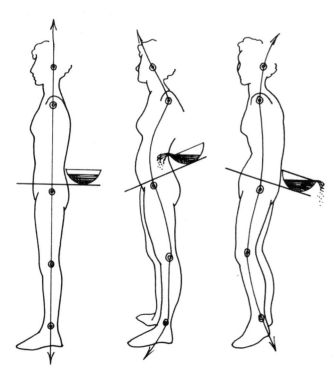

Figure 3

3. *Hips and Pelvic Girdle*

The pelvic girdle is like a cube (box) housing six sides. The two I refer to most frequently in my exercises are the front and back of the pelvic girdle: the pelvic triangle and the sacrum, as in figures 1 and 2.

The pelvic triangle is the front of the girdle and is formed by the two frontal hipbones and the pubic bone. The pelvic triangle must be level at all times. This means the hipbones must be in line with the pubic bone—perfectly vertical when you are upright and horizontal when you are prone.

The back of the pelvic girdle is the sacrum, and is the base of the spine. When the pelvic triangle is even, the sacrum is properly positioned and can do its job, which is to support the spine and cradle the abdomen. This job is especially noticeable when you are lying on your back. In the torso, only the flat shoulder blades and the sacrum should be making contact with the floor.

The other four parts of the pelvic girdle are the top (the waist where you hang your belt), the bottom (the perinium or crotch), the heads of the ischial bones (sit bones), and the two sides made up of two ilias (hipbones).

The mechanical purpose of the pelvic girdle is to provide an anchorage system. This consists of all the large paraspinal muscles of the spine—the abdominals, buttocks, and hamstrings. The upper hip area and a portion of the quadriceps muscle also attach to the pelvic girdle. The pelvis is a linkage system that allows the spinal column to connect with the lower extremity by way of the hip joints.

Perfect posture, as you know, starts with the feet, goes through the knees, and then must be upheld by the pelvic girdle—often where posture is lost. Most of the time, the girdle is too far back and produces a swayback; or it is too far forward.

I would like you to think of the pelvic girdle as a bowl filled with liquid. When it is perfectly balanced, as in figure 3, the liquid is contained. The most common imbalance is when the hips come before the pubic bone. The bowl is tipped, and the abdomen (liquid) falls out. This puts tremendous pressure on the lower back and often leads to pain and other problems. When the pubic bone is before the hips, the bowl is tipped on the other side, and the liquid is once again lost.

In all movements, it is essential to preserve and nurture the proper alignment of the pelvic girdle. If the pelvic cube is not balanced symmetrically in a squared-off position, it affects the four curves of the back. In the neutral position, the pubic bone is less than one-quarter of an inch behind the frontal hipbone. However, the majority of students I see, with their weak abdominals and backs, lack the awareness and ability to balance their pelvic girdles, so I emphasize, "the pubic bone to the pole" or "line up the pubic bone with the frontal hipbones" in the exercise instructions. For those who stand with the pubic bone forward, the pole presses so obviously they back off, bringing their pelvic girdle in balance.

Perfect balance in the pelvis ensures adequate space for the entire contents of the pelvic bowl, the viscera. It also decreases the chances of illness resulting from the stagnation of body fluids or the compression of nerves and organs.

With the American mania for playing with pain, the pelvic girdle is one of the most vulnerable areas. Americans continually attempt to touch their toes from a sitting position even if their backs, hips, and stomachs feel like an over-stuffed binding of a book, which will eventually break down.

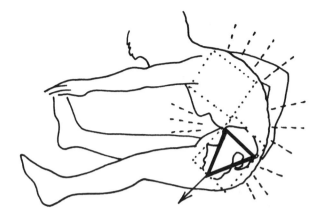

Figure 4

Does figure 4 look familiar to you? If this is the way you attempt a Sitting Forward Bend, with the pelvis tilted backward, you are stretching dangerously beyond the normal anatomical bounds. This position puts a great deal of stress on the lower back—more so if you forced yourself into the position by bouncing or pulling yourself down.

The rounded, hunched back is being forcibly pulled outward from its natural concaved position. It appears as a strained protrusion. (Feel it!) At the same time, imagine the oxygen-starved lungs in the sunken rib cage, not to mention the congested abdominal organs.

The correct figure 5 shows the pelvis squared off and anchored on the floor by the ischial bones. Notice that stretching is always done in straight lines. Imagine two lines from the extended heels through the middle toes. They should be parallel to each other. The kneecaps should point straight upward and be lifted toward the thighs. Sit as far forward as possible on the sit bones. The lumbar spine should attain a smooth groove and should not protrude outward. (Feel with your fingers.) All this is done before you bend forward. It is called aligning the body for a Forward Bend. Observe the symmetrical balance between the shoulder and pelvic girdle.

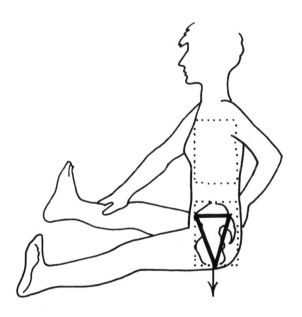

Figure 5

Direct your energy both down the legs to the extended heels and back toward the rooted ischial bones. Simultaneously, direct your energy upward from the ischial bones to the top of the head. You will find that by applying the principles of elongation and by concaving the spine upward, you will be able to use this natural placement of the spine to move upward and forward as a ratchet, as in figure 6. For the "ideal" back, don't forget to breathe in rhythm.

I know that for most of you this is an elusive goal. Because you are very tight in the hamstrings and hips, sitting on the floor with an aligned spine is almost an impossibility. That is why the first exercise in this chapter is Sitting Up on the Ischial Bones at stairs.

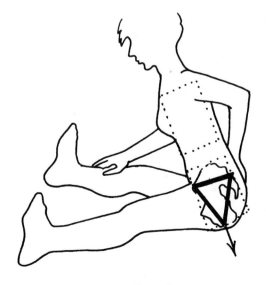

Figure 6

Another exercise that highly abuses the pelvic girdle is The Plow. Because of the status of most people's bodies, I rarely recommend even attempting this exercise. Most people need a great deal of preparation and the direction of a fine teacher before doing The Plow correctly. However, if you currently have The Plow in your exercise program and intend to keep it there, I have described how to perform it *correctly* in the last exercise of this chapter.

SITTING UP ON THE ISCHIAL BONES

Props

1. A stairway.
2. A leg of a table.
3. A tie or belt.
4. A stack of books.

Body Placement

1. Sit with the ischial bones on the edge of the second step, as in figure 1b. With the knees bent and the left hand pulling the left knee, take the right hand and feel to check if the spine is protruding incorrectly, as in figure 1a. In the correct position, it should be recessed into a continual, smooth groove throughout its length, as in figure 2a.
2. If you are sitting up too high, your spine will be rutted too deep. To acquire the smooth groove, lower your ischium to one of the three sitting positions in figures 2b, 3, or 4.
3. If you have hyperextended knees, make sure you don't just let your legs hang and lock back. Keep them eased and the knee-caps raised toward the thighs. If your hips are open enough, the best position for you is figure 4.
4. Carefully consider steps 1-3 and sit in a position that is right for you.

Technique

1. Inhale and elongate the spine. While extending the sternum, roll your shoulders back and down to create a blade squeeze.
2. Exhale and feed the spine deeper into the body, as you ground your ischium straight down.
3. Inhale and repeat the elongation and extension.
4. While exhaling, secure your alignment and a firm foundation on those ischial bones. Work to straighten the legs, as in figure 2b.

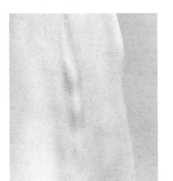

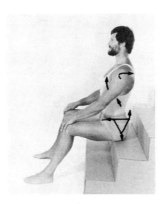

a
INCORRECT

b

Figure 1

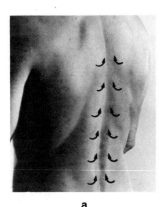

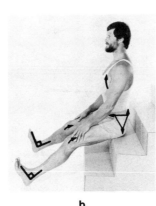

a

b

Figure 2

5. Hold the breath out for the count of six, as you continue to rotate the pelvic girdle forward and follow with the spine.

6. Repeat steps 1-5 five more times. Rest. You now have found your ischial bones and know why they are called "sit bones!"

Variation 1

1. Sit close so the post (leg) of a table is between your legs, as in figure 3.

2. Wrap a belt around the post and hold both straps in your left hand. This frees the right to feel the back. When you "know" your back, you can hold each strap in separate hands, as in figure 3.

3. The leverage you need for the elongation and extension is attained by the pull on the belt and by making sure the elbows start beside and work behind the ribs.

4. The number of books you sit on will depend on what you need to acquire a long, smooth groove.

5. Follow Technique steps 1-6.

6. As you become more flexible, remove the books one by one.

Variation 2

1. Now that you know how to sit squarely on the floor, with your ischium grounded and your back in a smooth groove, as in figure 4, you may proceed.

2. Follow Technique steps 1-6. Work at pressing your legs down into the floor by extending the heels, raising the knee-caps, and keeping the thighs down. This gives the internal lift for the pelvis to rotate forward, aligning the body and enabling it to move forward.

Tips

1. The action in the legs plays an important part in the correct rotation of the hips. The angle of the foot, knees, and ball of the foot is extended. The kneecaps are raised toward the thighs, which tightens them. This total action protects the hyperextended knees.

2. Keeping the elbows at or behind the ribs helps tremendously in the elongation and extension of the spine.

3. Don't just pull the belt. It is acting as leverage so the body can align itself.

Benefits

This exercise aligns and frees the pelvic girdle and each disc in the vertebral column. It also stretches the legs.

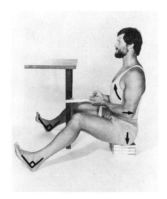

Figure 3

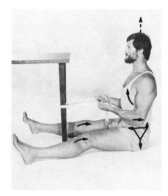

Figure 4

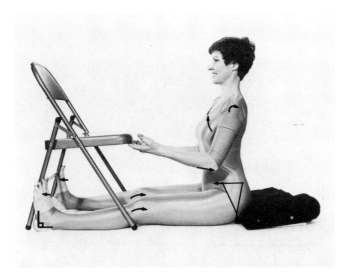

Figure 1

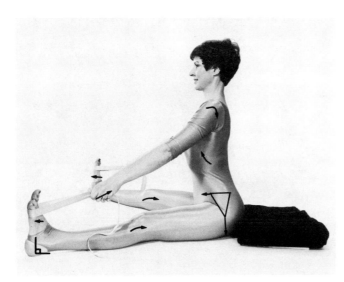

Figure 2

SITTING FORWARD BEND

Props

1. A chair.
2. Two belts.
3. Books or blankets.

Body Placement

1. Review the previous exercise, Sitting Up on the Ischial Bones, to understand the best position for the alignment of your pelvic girdle and spine.
2. To sit as in figure 1:
    a. Sit straight up on your ischial bones with a book or blanket under you.
    b. Slide your ischial bones just off the edge of the books or blanket. Lean the buttocks, shin, and muscle on the books or blanket. This helps in the rotation of the pelvis.
    c. Pull up the chair so the back two legs meet the feet. Press the heels and balls of the feet into the legs of the chair.
    d. Use your hands, bending the elbows, to pull the underpart or sides of the chair for leverage.
3. To sit as in figure 2:
    a. With the legs wide apart, loop two belts around the balls of the feet. Make the loop small enough so your arms can be straight. The spine should make a smooth groove.
    b. Slide your ischial bones just off the edge of the books or blanket.
4. To sit as in figure 3:
    a. Position the legs hip-distance apart or together and loop a belt around the balls of the feet so your arms can be straight.
    b. Slide your ischial bones just off the edge of the books or blanket.

5. To sit as in figure 4:
   a. Legs are hip-distance apart or together.
   b. Keep your heels on the floor. Grab the balls of the feet with your fingers for leverage to draw the body forward.
   c. As your flexibility increases, you can grab your wrist behind your feet and work up your arm.

Technique

1. As you inhale, elongate and extend the front of the body. Ground yourself on your ischial bones.
2. While exhaling, secure your alignment (smooth groove) and firm foundation (being grounded).
3. Hold the breath out and count to six, as you continue to rotate the frontal hipbones forward. Follow with advancing the spine.
4. Repeat steps 1-3 five more times. Rest.

Tips

1. These sitting forward positions can be helpful only if you execute them at your own level of ability.
2. Remember, it's not what you do that counts, it's how well you are doing it that's important.
3. Check your back periodically with one hand to make sure you maintain your smooth groove (recessed spine). As you advance forward, your smooth groove will disappear; but the frontal hipbones should stay forward.

Benefits

In a more advanced way, this exercise aligns and frees the pelvic girdle and discs along the vertebral column. It also stretches the legs.

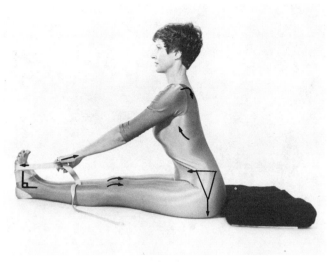

Figure 3

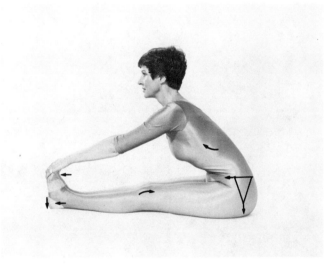

Figure 4

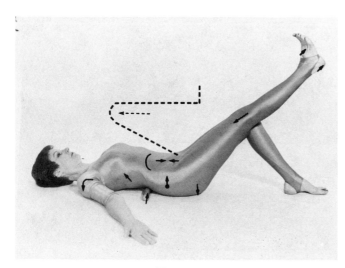

Figure 1

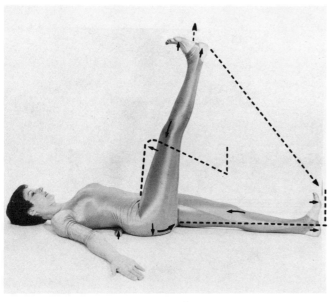

Figure 2

SUPINE LEG RAISE

Props

1. A one-inch thick pole or magazine (rolled up).
2. A belt.

Body Placement

1. Read the discussion on Abdominal Muscles (section IV, chapter 4) and review the exercises to understand the importance of having the waist off the floor.
2. To do the Leg Raise as in figures 1 and 2, lie down with the pole under your waist and keep your knees bent.
3. To do the Leg Raise as in figure 3:
   a. Do this Variation only if you can do step 2 with your spine off the pole.
   b. Lie down. Wrap the belt around the ball of your right foot and hold it with your left hand.
   c. With the right leg straight up, place your right thumb over the muscle at the hipbone. Pull the muscle out to the side and away from you, while drawing your ischial bones closer together. By sensing this action, you are aligning your pelvic girdle.
   d. Do *not* advance the leg by opening the hip out to the side.
   e. You don't need the pole because the back does lower slightly; but the spine should *not* press into the floor. You are continually recessing it into the body with the sacrum being your base.
4. To do the Leg Raise as in figure 4:
   a. Bend your knees and wrap a belt across both balls of both feet.
   b. Straighten your legs up vertically with the waist off the floor and the sacrum grounded.

Technique

1. Inhale as you elongate the spine with the sacrum as your base. Stretch up and out of your waist, which is off the pole or floor.
2. While exhaling, contract your abdomen and apply a blade squeeze to flatten your shoulders.
3. To do the Leg Raise as in figure 1:
   a. Inhale and bend the knee to the chest.
   b. Exhale and straighten the leg out to the left thigh.

c. Hold the position for five counts.

d. Repeat the breathing and motion rhythm by bringing the knee to the chest.

4. To do the Leg Raise as in figure 2:

   a. Inhale and bend the knee to the chest.

   b. Exhale and straighten the leg up high and lower it to one inch off the floor.

   c. Hold the position for a count of five.

   d. Repeat while bending the knee to the chest.

5. To do the Leg Raise as in figure 3:

   a. Inhale and elongate the spine, using the thumb for leverage.

   b. Exhale and push with your thumb to anchor on your sacrum. Contract the abdomen.

   c. Hold your control as you advance the right leg, while pressing the left leg into the floor.

   d. Repeat the breathing and motion rhythm.

6. To do the Leg Raise as in figure 4:

   a. Inhale. Elongate the spine and extend the chest, using straight arms with the belt as leverage.

   b. Exhale and contract your abdomen, dipping the tailbone downward.

   c. Hold your firm foundation as you advance the legs forward.

   d. Repeat the breathing and motion rhythm.

7. Continue the breathing and motion rhythm with the Leg Raise that is right for you.

8. Repeat the cycle five times. Rest and repeat with the left leg, as in figures 1-3.

Tips

1. Make sure in all four Leg Raises that the waist does *not* press into the pole or floor. You want to maintain the natural lumbar curve.

2. Make sure you ground the leg by dipping the tailbone downward before and while advancing the leg.

3. Dipping the tailbone downward secures the pelvic triangle and keeps your buttocks from rolling off the floor when advancing the leg.

Benefits

This exercise is an excellent stretch for the hamstrings. It strengthens the control of the pelvic girdle and makes the hip socket stronger.

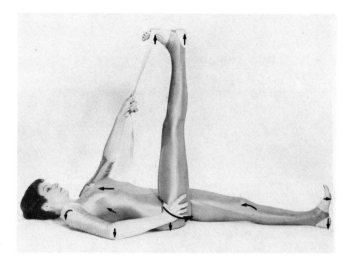

Figure 3

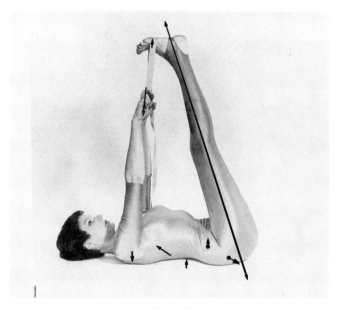

Figure 4

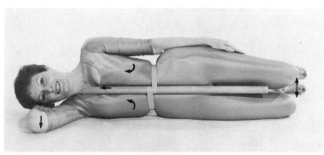

Figure 1

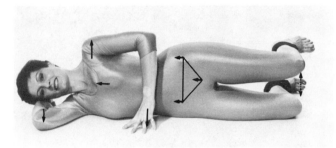

Figure 2

RECLINED SIDE BALANCE

Props

1. A set of three-pound ankle weights.
2. A 2½-foot pole or the attachment from a vacuum.
3. A nylon belt with two rings to slide closed.

Body Placement

It would be to your advantage to learn this exercise and its Variations by wearing the pole tied *very* tightly with a belt. Once you attain the alignment and control, you can do without the pole.

1. Lie down on your right side. Bend your right elbow and make a fist with your hand, placing your head on the curled little finger.
2. Place the fingertips of your left hand on the floor at your waist for support.
3. To align the upper body, press your fingers into the floor and extend the chest to create a blade squeeze.
4. Bend the legs at the knees, forming a right angle at the knees and heels, as in figure 1.

Technique

1. Inhale and elongate the spine with the sternum on the pole.
2. Exhale and contract the abdomen away from the pole, while rotating the pubic bone to the pole, as in figure 1.
3. Lift the left knee level with the hip. Hold this alignment for the count of six. The sternum, ribs, hips, pubic bone, and knees should be in a straight line.
4. Rest and repeat five times.

Variation 1, figure 2

1. Repeat Technique steps 1-3; but use the ankle weights.
2. On the exhalation, maintain the alignment to the pole. While you work the left thigh back, keep your pubic bone on the pole, as in figure 2.
3. Hold this position for a count of six. Rest and repeat five times. Then turn over and repeat the cycle on the left side. Good work! Looked easy, didn't it!

Variation 2, figure 3

1. Repeat Technique steps 1-3 with the ankle weights.
2. On the exhalation, maintain the alignment to the pole and straighten out the right leg.
3. With a contracted abdomen and the pubic bone to the pole, raise and lower the leg ten times.
4. Rest and repeat two more times *only* if you can maintain contact with the pole and balance.
5. Turn over onto the left side and repeat the cycle.

Variation 3, figure 4

1. You can do this with or without weights.
2. Repeat Technique steps 1-3.
3. On the exhalation, maintain alignment to the pole. While you straighten out both legs, balance on the side of your hip and raise up both legs.
4. Hold this balance, take your left hand off and balance on your hip. Keep your knees, pubic bone, hips, and ribs in line.
5. Hold for the count of six. Rest. Repeat five times. Then turn onto the left side and repeat the cycle.

Tips

1. As I have said, start off using the pole — it's like having me at home with you to keep you in line. As you acquire control, you can do without the pole.
2. You can do all four exercises in sequence. Then turn on the other side and repeat with figures 1-4.
3. Keep the arm that's at your waist up close so you won't tilt over.

Benefits

This exercise firms the hips and thighs. It also tones the abdominal muscles and promotes balance.

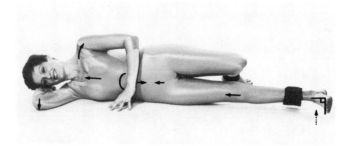

Figure 3

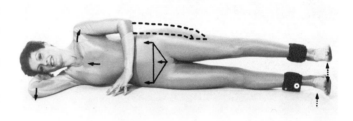

Figure 4

THE PLOW

The Plow is the most misused exercise. People swing their legs over their heads, while being destructive to their neck and while compressing their blood vessels to the brain and spinal cord. The Plow strains the whole length of the spine, tearing the ligaments in the back and adding injury to the sciatic nerve. Need I say more?

For the fitness of the average person, this exercise is too complicated. I don't feel one needs to accomplish it. My Total Fitness Daily Dozen Routine (section V, chapter 1) gives you a well-rounded program without The Plow.

I recommend this exercise *only* for the advanced student and *only* with the following directions.

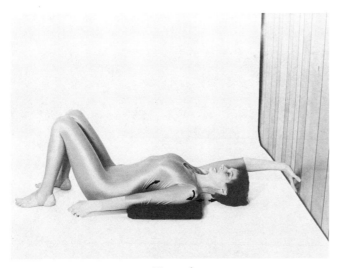

Figure 1

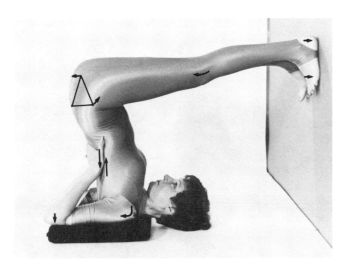

a

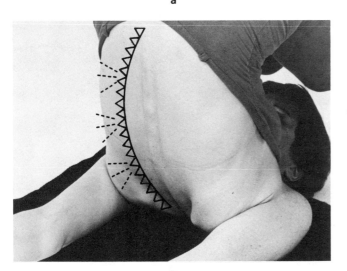

b
Figure 2
INCORRECT

Props

1. A wall.
2. A belt tied to loop the width of the shoulders. If the shoulders are tight, the belt must be wider. Once in position with the belt on, you must feel weight on the upper arms, not just on the shoulders.
3. Four to six inches of firm (army) blankets folded to fit from the elbows to the shoulders. Both the elbows and shoulders should be firmly on the same level for support.

Body Placement

1. Take the time to adjust the height of your shoulders, using the blankets. This will keep your throat and neck soft and comfortable throughout the exercise.
2. Line up the blankets with the folded edge in a sharp even line, facing the wall.
3. Place your back on top of the blankets with your head on the floor at the distance where your fingers touch the wall, as in figure 1. If it's uncomfortable for your neck, you either don't need as much support or you need more. Remove or add one layer at a time. If it continues to be unpleasant, you are probably pressing your cervical (neck) spine out and into the floor. When on top of the blankets, walk your shoulders together to create a blade squeeze. Bring the cervical spine up into the neck. You are now balancing on your upper arms. Your neck should feel better.
4. Lift up your buttocks so you can slide your arms through the belt. Stop just above your elbows.
5. Rock up and back, get the feet to the wall, and straighten your legs. Your toes and heels should be flat against the wall and your legs parallel to the floor.
   a. With the belt above the elbows, clasp your hands and walk your shoulders together. Create a tight blade squeeze. You should be off your neck and up on your upper arms and shoulders, as in figure 2a.
   b. If it is still uncomfortable in your throat and neck, you are too far away from the wall.
   c. Come down and start over, carefully adjusting your distance.

Technique

1. Inhale, still clasping your hands. Turn your elbows in and shrug your shoulders down away from your ears, about one inch from the sharp edge of your blankets, as in figure 2a.
2. Exhale as you lift up your hips to elongate and straighten your back. Make a right angle with the legs, as in figure 3a. Your spine should be recessed and completely off the blankets.

3. Inhale, bending at the elbows and placing your hands as high as possible toward the shoulders, as in figure 2a. Move the skin of your neck and shoulder area out of the way in the direction of the waist so your hands ultimately grip a taut back. Don't push your elbows into the belt. Try to draw them away. The belt keeps your elbows in line with your shoulders and your upper back lifted.

4. Feel your spine with one hand to make sure it doesn't feel like the one in figure 2b. It should feel like the one in figure 3b.

5. Exhale, pushing your heels away from the wall with the toes. Raise your kneecaps toward the thighs, while concaving the spine. Work your hands further onto the back and just under the shoulder blades, as in figure 3a.

6. In this position, inhale and extend the sternum, while lifting and elongating the spine.

7. While exhaling, further concave the back as you lift up. Extend and move your ischial bones toward each other and to the ceiling. Notice the relief in your neck and breathing.

8. Repeat steps 6 and 7 three times with the suggested breathing rhythm. When the balance is achieved, you will find your spine is recessed and your weight is directly on top of your shoulders and elbows, firmly pressed down onto the blankets.

9. To come down, exhale slowly and walk your toes down the wall *without* rounding your back or changing the placement of your hips, as in figure 4. Go down only as far as you can maintain the alignment of the hips and back. This is your spot to work on the wall. Inhale when ready to come down and carefully come out of it on exhalation.

Tips

1. I have given you all the instructions. As you can see, there are a lot of details. The important thing I want you to remember is: It is not worth doing if you have any discomfort in the neck, head, or throat.

2. Take time to adjust your props and place them the correct distance from the wall for your leg length and flexibility.

3. There is a continual action of lifting up toward the ceiling. Press your upper arm and shoulders down as the base from which the lift comes. Do not lean forward or backward.

Benefits

When done correctly, this exercise is an excellent massage and strengthener for the spinal column. It stretches the hamstrings and helps to equalize the thyroid.

• This exercise is recommended to be done *only* under the guidance of a trained instructor.

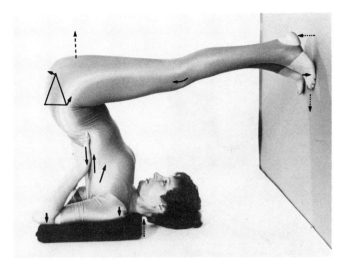

a

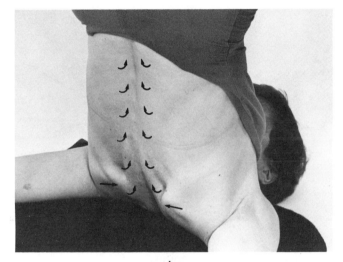

b

Figure 3

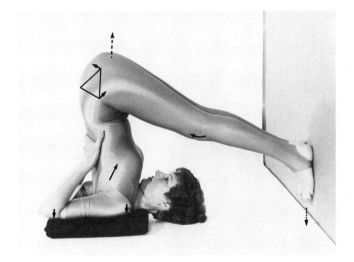

Figure 4

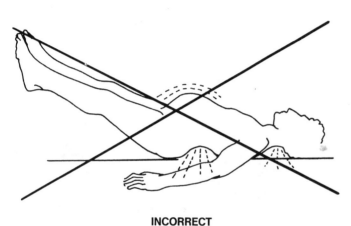

INCORRECT

4. Abdominal Muscles

The abdominal muscles are among the most misunderstood groups of muscles in the body and probably the most abused in exercise programs. These are supportive muscles whose function is to brace the spine, chest, and pelvis and hold your organs in place.

Ida P. Rolf, the well-known creator of corrective muscle massage, observes that physical training programs are preoccupied with the rectus abdominis. In their attempt to "strengthen" the abdominals, they prescribe repetitious sit-ups. Active gym people are so proud of the definition of their abdominal wall that they invite you to punch it to test its hardness, saying, "See, all muscle!" Yes, it is all muscle; but it is rigid, tense, and protruded muscle, which weakens their lumbar spines and sets them up for future pain and problems.

The poor gym people have built their exercise programs around the misconception that a hard abdomen means one with so-called strength. They have built up a mass of too much unyielding muscle. Hardening of the abdominal muscles means that the muscular layers have hypertrophied together and are less able to accept the rapid lengthening and shortening, which is essential to healthy muscle functioning. True strength is derived from the interaction of and balance between the agonist (front contraction) and the antagonist (back relax-stretch). In well-executed activity, the reciprocal directional pull and contraction of the agonist-antagonist is responsible for correct balance and strength. True strength is *not* hardening; true strength is resilience, adaptability, and stability. Its character is elasticity.

Doing six double Leg Lifts or thirty Sit-Ups a day shortens and hardens abdominal muscles that are often too short. This further upsets the agonist-antagonist balance. What Sit-Ups really do is to create a tightened psoas muscle. The psoas is crucial in determining the amount of tilt the pelvis takes. When the psoas is too tight, the pelvis will assume a forward tilt and will create the characteristic swayback condition—tension in the lower back and an excessively protruding belly.

The psoas attaches to the belly side of all five lumbar vertebrae, then descends downward in the pelvis, crosses the hip joint, and connects to the inner edge of the thighbone, as in figure 1. This muscle initiates walking by lifting up the thighbone.

The muscles that act in opposition to the psoas are the abdominals. For correct positioning of the pelvis, the psoas and abdominals should have equal tone, flexibility, and strength, as in figure 2a. For example, if the psoas is short and tight, a swayback posture occurs (a usual condition in our society because of our sitting habits), which shows the imbalance between the psoas and abdominals, as in figure 2b. So pay close attention to the instruction for aligning the pelvic triangle with abdominal control, which can rectify the swayback condition.

I frequently see the signs that the psoas is not balanced in athletes who come in because of "back or groin pain." They are active so they don't necessarily have pot bellies. However, their pelvises are tilted forward, lumbar spines are hyperextended, and chests are dropped. This causes the pain.

It seems like the whole country is trying to tighten and harden its stomach—a very laudable goal but, often, a misdirected effort. Remember, tightening the stomach *does not flatten* it! When doing the classical sit-ups, one strains the abdominals out—jamming the insides (organs) down and outward, creating that hard, protruding abdomen.

If this sounds odd, think about it and check for yourself. When people exercise with the abdomen popped out, they are encouraging a hard, protruded abdomen. Also, they are working to press the spine on the floor and are tipping the pelvis. This rolls the tailbone upward, shortens the muscle, and encourages a protruded abdomen. To tip the pelvis, you might look flat. However, you are deceiving yourself by taking only the abdominals for a swim inward. Be honest. When you exert any effort, don't they pop? Remember, you are also inviting lower back problems.

I am very aware of the "tip pelvis technique" that rotates the pelvis forward at the expense of the spine's natural curve. I used it myself in the past; but I noticed I was getting a protruded abdomen with no added strength, and I was experiencing tension in the neck. This prompted me to study how the body was meant to be used. I found that one should keep the natural lumbar curve and anchor one's balance on the sacrum.

Just how much curve? I solved it by using a one-inch thick pole to keep the spine in neutral—not too arched up or rolled toward the floor. The pelvic girdle should be level. Throughout this book you will read "keep your pelvic triangle level." To monitor this position, I encourage my students to place the heels of their hands on the hipbones with their fingers on the pubic bone. This keeps you aware of not popping your abdominals and of levelling the pelvic girdle. Try it. The pole is comfortable under the waist at all times. In my seven years of teaching this technique, I have not found a back that the one-inch pole didn't fit once we aligned the pelvic girdle and upper body. I know there are exceptions; but for those, I recommend using a smaller pole. I don't want any of you to use excuses. Give it a good try—it works!

Another example to help you contract the abdominals correctly is to think of two upholstered buttons. One is in the center of the sacrum, and the other one is centered between the navel and the pubic bone just above the sacrum. As you contract the abdominals and work in the exercise, continue to tighten the

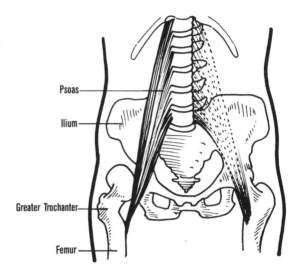

Figure 1

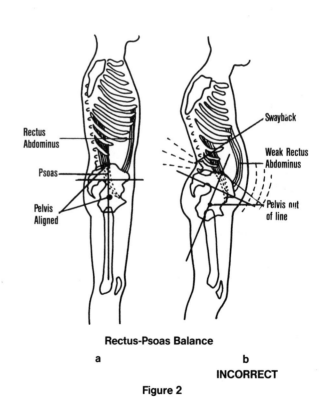

Rectus-Psoas Balance

a   b
INCORRECT

Figure 2

string that pulls the two buttons closer together. You have to concentrate all the time on using the abdominals correctly. They might seem to have a mind of their own; but, remember, *you* are in control of those abdominals.

Don't use the excuse your stomach is too big to work correctly. All the abdominal exercises work from inside, no matter what shape the stomach is in. As you perform the exercises regularly and correctly, you will feel the deep work going on inside. Soon you will see the results of your efforts—a flat and firm silhouette.

For psychological as well as physiological advantage, I want you to probe the abdominal muscles with your fingers. You'll find that they soften as they relax and harden as they come into action by contracting on your exhalation. Even when you're trained, probing to find the contracted abdomen will reassure you that you are doing the exercise correctly.

I am not interested in your executing my exercises to an advanced degree immediately. It's better if you exercise to your own personal limit of effort. I define this limit as a slight over-load; that is, to the edge of your capacity. But you're the one who gauges that effort in terms of your own resources. Check with your probing fingers to see that you are keeping a *flat* and firm abdominal wall and that your pelvic triangle is level. When you feel your abdomen strain outward or pop, go back to the point where the effort will be *moderately difficult, but correct.* That's a good position for you.

Now that your position for moderate exertion has been well-defined, your level of exertion will improve with your condition; but be more concerned with getting the most value from each position, rather than with advancing to more difficult ones. You're getting just as much value out of the first position when you're in poor condition as you are from the last position when you're in good condition. The exercises are presented in a graduated manner. Do not rush through the material. It's the quality of the control that you can maintain that counts, not the number of variations and repetitions that you can do. I always say, "Quality, not Quantity—have Bodysense!"

SACRUM AND ABDOMINAL PRESS

Props

1. Fold a facecloth in half three times. Place it under your sacrum, as in figure 1a.
2. Place a one-inch thick pole under your waist, as in figure 1b.

Body Placement

1. Lie down. Tuck your buttocks away toward your thighs, balancing the sacrum in the facecloth.
2. Using your elbows, lift your chest to squeeze the shoulder blades flat.
3. With your hands, align your pelvic triangle. Make the pole comfortable.

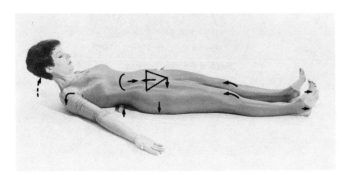

a

b

Figure 1

Technique

1. Inhale and elongate the spine upward. Anchor yourself on the sacrum.
2. While exhaling, contract your abdomen and raise your head, as in figure 1b.
3. Hold the breath out for six counts and continue to press the abdomen down onto the sacrum.
4. Rest your head.
5. Repeat ten times.

Variation 1, figure 2

1. With the facecloth and pole still under you, draw the soles of the feet together with the knees out to the side, as in figure 2.
2. Repeat Technique steps 1-5. Open your legs, relax the hip area, and work the abdominals correctly.

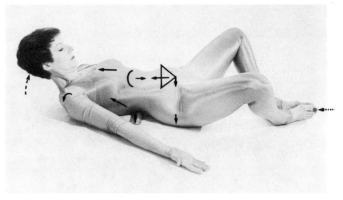

Figure 2

Variation 2, figure 3

1. Put your knees together and straighten the right leg. Slide your left ankle so it is at the right leg's mid-calf, as in figure 3.
2. Repeat Technique steps 1-3. During step 3, raise the right leg just one inch off the floor for six counts.
3. Rest.
4. Repeat the cycle five more times, alternating the legs.

Variation 3, figure 4

1. With both the legs straight, feet flexed, and heels extended, repeat Technique steps 1-3.
2. During step 3, raise the left leg just one inch off the floor, as shown in figure 4.
3. Use the right leg as leverage to maintain a level triangle and tighten the abdominals.
4. Rest. Surprised that you could get such a good inward feeling?
5. Repeat the cycle five more times, alternating the legs.

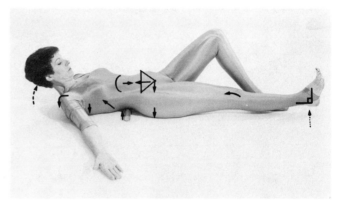

Figure 3

Tips

1. At no time should your abdominal muscles pop or press outward. There should be a feeling of shrinking, contracting, and flattening, while executing these exercises.
2. Once you have mastered the exercises, remove the facecloth.
3. Raise only your head and one leg at a time one inch off the floor—no more!
4. These are graduated exercises. Work at your own level.
5. As the exercise becomes effortless, add ankle weights.

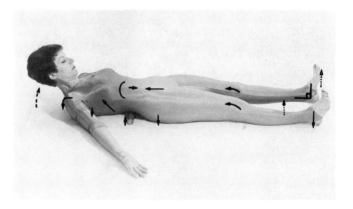

Figure 4

Rhythm

1. Inhale to get ready.
2. Exhale 50 percent of your breath, while contracting your abdomen. Then continue to expel the remaining breath, while executing the exercise.
3. Hold the position for a count of six without inhaling.
4. Inhale and rest.
5. Repeat the cycle.

Benefits

The abdominals are flattened, firmed, and strengthened. The back becomes stronger and is protected. The neck is also strengthened.

SACRUM BALANCE AT WALL

Props

1. A one-inch thick pole under your waist.

Body Placement

1. Lie down. Place your feet on the wall so your legs form a right angle. Balance on the sacrum.
2. Place the balls of the feet on the wall but keep the heels off, as in figure 1.
3. Using your elbows, lift your chest to squeeze the shoulder blades flat.

Technique

1. Inhale and elongate your ribs up out of your waist. Anchor on the sacrum.
2. Exhale and contract your abdomen. While flexing at the ankle, draw the ball of the right foot away from the wall without moving your knee or leg, as in figure 2.
3. Hold your breath out for a count of six. Apply a slight push with the left foot to further aid in contracting the abdominals tighter.
4. Return your foot and repeat with the left one.
5. Repeat the cycle as long as you can keep the pelvic triangle level and the abdomen from popping, while lifting the foot off the wall.

Variation 1, figure 3

1. Keep both balls of the feet to the wall, as in figure 1.

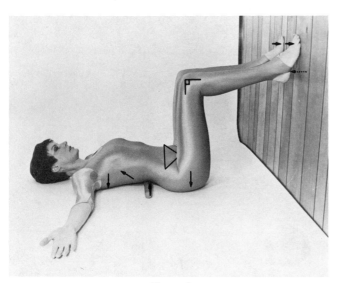

Figure 1

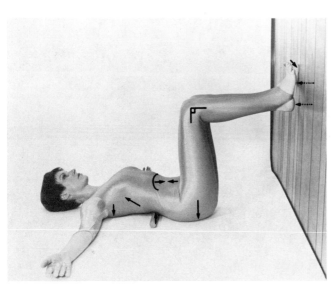

Figure 2

2. Repeat Technique steps 1-3. After a slight push with the left foot, slowly lift it one inch off the wall. The abdomen should remain flat and firm. Hold.
3. Return the feet to the wall. Repeat the cycle, alternating the feet.
4. Repeat ten more times.

Variation 2, figure 4

1. This is a graduated series. Repeat Variation 1, steps 1 and 2.
2. Working your feet down the wall, create a more difficult leverage. Stop at the point where your abdomen loses control.
3. Work just above that level until you gain the proper strength to go further. This might be as far as you work for awhile.
4. When you reach the floor, rest.
5. Inhale. While exhaling, really contract those abdominals. Keep your spine comfortably on the pole, as you lift the feet off the floor. If you can do this without popping your stomach, you can work this exercise from the floor without the wall.
6. Repeat ten more times from the floor or wall.

Tips

1. The pole keeps you in neutral. Don't press it hard or arch way off.
2. Lift your feet only when you have completed the exhalation.
3. Remember, it's not how far you go but the quality of abdominal strength that counts.
4. If you have mastered the whole series without the abdomen popping, you may repeat the series with raising your head. Only then, repeat with three-pound ankle weights.

Benefits

The abdominals become flattened and firmed. The back is strengthened and the spine is aligned.

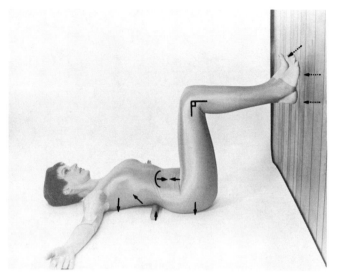

Figure 3

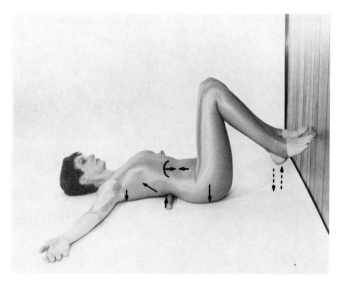

Figure 4

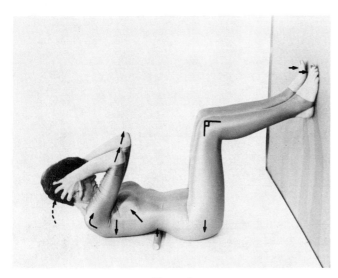

Figure 1

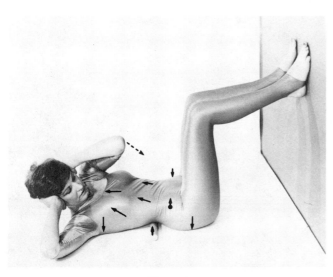

Figure 2

SACRUM BALANCE WITH ROLL-UP

Props

1. A one-inch thick pole under your waist.
2. A wall.

Body Placement

1. Lie down. Place your feet on the wall so your legs form a right angle.
2. The feet stay flat on the wall.
3. Place your hands to cup your ears, with your elbows toward the knees, as in figure 1.
4. Dip your tailbone to the floor to properly anchor on your sacrum. Don't roll your buttocks upward.

Technique

1. While inhaling, elongate your ribs up out of your waist. Anchor on your sacrum with the pole comfortably under your back.
2. While exhaling, contract your abdomen and draw only your head and the tops of your shoulders off the floor, as in figure 1.
3. Hold your breath out for six counts, while dipping your tailbone into the floor. Push slightly with your feet to further contract the abdomen. Still keeping off the pole, balance on the center of the sacrum.
4. Lower your head and shoulders. Repeat until you can accomplish keeping the pelvic triangle level and the abdomen from popping.

Variation 1, figure 2

1. Repeat Technique steps 1-3. Upon holding your breath out, maintain your anchored abdominals. Cross your left elbow over to the right side, keeping the ribs out of the waist, as in figure 2.

2. Dip your tailbone down and keep the pelvic triangle level, even while twisting the upper body.
3. Rest your head. Repeat with the opposite elbow.
4. Repeat ten more times.

Variation 2, figure 3

1. Repeat Variation 1, steps 1 and 2.
2. While reaching over with your left elbow and feeling secure in the abdominal balance, lift the right foot one inch off the wall, as in figure 3.
3. Hold the balance for a count of six. Still remain off the pole.
4. Rest your head and foot. Repeat with the opposite side.
5. Repeat ten more times.

Variation 3, figure 4

1. Repeat Variation 2, steps 1-3.
2. With your balance properly secured, lift your other foot just one inch off the wall, as in figure 4.
3. Rest your head and feet. Repeat with the opposite side.
4. Repeat ten more times.

Tips

1. This is a graduated exercise. So remember, it's the quality of the doing that counts.
2. As the exercise becomes effortless, you may add ankle weights first and then do more repetitions.
3. The pole should remain comfortable at all times.

Benefits

This exercise strengthens the neck, abdominals, and back. It is particularly helpful in keeping those with pot bellies from being swayback.

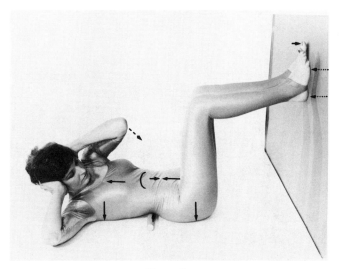

Figure 3

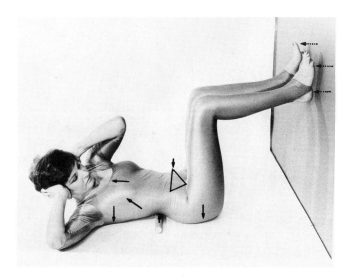

Figure 4

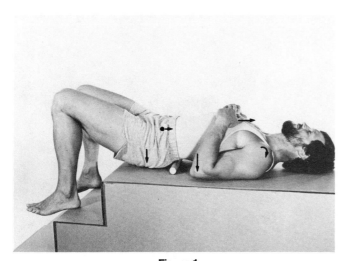

Figure 1

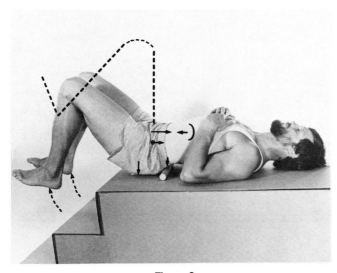

Figure 2

SACRUM BALANCE AT STAIRS

Props

1. A one-inch thick pole under your waist.

Body Placement

1. Lie down at the top of the stairs. Place your buttocks at the edge of the step and feet on the next step, as in figure 1.
2. Concentrate on keeping close to the pole as the leverage gets more difficult.
3. Using your elbows, lift your chest to squeeze the shoulder blades flat.

Technique

1. Inhale and elongate the spine, while anchoring on your sacrum.
2. While exhaling, tightly contract the abdominals and ribs as you completely expel your breath. Keep a *slight* pressure on the pole as you raise your knees directly over your hips, as in figure 2. Hope you didn't think this was going to be easy!

Variation 1, figure 3

1. Repeat Technique steps 1 and 2. Inhale and breathe out completely. With your abdomen contracted, slowly lower your feet to the first step, as in figure 3.
2. Do not pull away from the pole.
3. Rest on the step. Inhale and repeat the full cycle. Not as easy as it looks, is it?
4. Repeat ten more times.

Variation 2, figure 4

CAUTION: Unless the above is done with ease, do *not* attempt this variation.

1. Place your feet on the second step, as in figure 4.
2. Apply Technique steps 1 and 2. With complete abdominal control, raise two feet off the second step, while drawing the knees above the hips.
3. Rest and inhale.
4. Exhale and slowly lower the legs again to the second step. Rest and inhale while on the second step. This is one cycle. Good, you made it! Make sure you keep contracting the abdominals toward the pole.
5. Repeat ten times.

Tips

1. Your abdominals should feel worked—contracted inward but *not* strained outward.
2. The back consistently remains near the pole so it will not be strained.
3. If you can complete this exercise correctly, add three-pound ankle weights.

Benefits

This exercise is an excellent firmer for the abdominals. It also strengthens the thoracic and lumbar areas of the back.

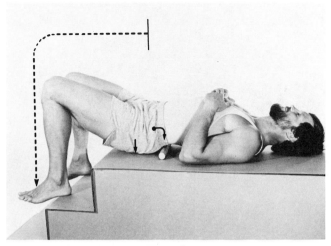

Figure 3

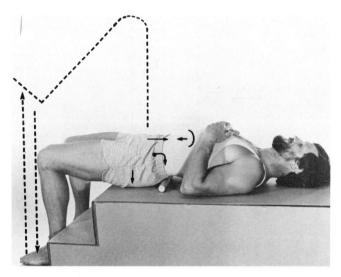

Figure 4

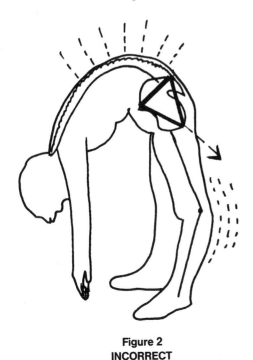

Cervical
Vertebrae

Thoracic
Vertebrae

Lumbar
Vertebrae

Sacral
Vertebrae

Acetabulum
(Ball Socket)

Figure 1

Figure 2
INCORRECT

5. The Back

The average spine is about twenty-seven inches in length. The spine has four normal curves: cervical (neck), thoracic (rib level), lumbar (below the ribs), and sacral (the curve at the top of the buttocks at the base of the spine).

The curves of the spine are formed by the different shapes and thicknesses of the individual vertebra, which are separated and cushioned by discs of cartilage and water. Any permanent alteration in one curve will affect the curves above or below.

The weight and stress of the entire body passes through each vertebra. When people overstretch, tug, or lift, using their spines in the manner shown in figure 2, they are overstraining and putting undue pressure in the lower lumbar area. Our lifestyle adds to the tendency to round the back in the way we sit, sleep, and drive. Continual stretching with the rounded back only reinforces this tendency and the ensuing problems.

Between the bones of the spine there are discs, hydraulic "shock absorbers," that allow for movement and compression. They account for the shape of the back and for one-fourth of its length. *As we approach thirty years of age, the blood supply to the discs retracts because we are fully mature. From then on, nourishment has to come from movement.* Fluids are drawn in and flushed out of the discs as we flex, extend, and twist the spine. Now, more than ever, since the fitness craze is spreading and injuries are increasing from improper exercises, the discs aren't getting properly nourished because they are compressed. So degeneration begins. The discs start to shrink and lose their elasticity, becoming more easily torn. As you get older, if you do not exercise properly and elongate your spine, the discs will start to shrink. This has a lot of possible ramifications, such as herniation and pressure on the sciatic nerve root. Having sway-back puts continual pressure on the back of the discs; this may eventually degenerate, with pain to follow.

When a disc is damaged or ruptured, a gelatinous matter oozes from it, and severe pain is caused because of the pressure on the spinal nerve roots, as in figure 3. For the health of the back, stretching is essential to lengthen the ligaments encasing the discs. This lengthening can allow the discs to return to a more plump, fuller state. Stretching creates more space between the vertebrae, which deters the flattening of the discs.

To ensure the safety of the back, the spine must be straight. The four normal curvatures of the spinal column allow optimal movement when stretched and elongated within their range of motion. The problem with most spines is that one or more of the curves becomes exaggerated, which throws everything off.

The spine is at its most extended position when it has its normal curves; although, the exact angle of the curves can differ from person to person. So, let's make sure you preserve the spinal column to your unique alignment.

Bend over with your back rounded and with legs straight, while placing your fingers on the back of your waist. You will probably feel the bones of your back poking up, making bumps, as in figure 4. Keeping your fingers on the bumps, bend your knees and lift your buttocks and ischial bones (sit bones) toward the ceiling, as in figure 7. The bumps should disappear into a smooth groove, as in figure 5. If this is not possible, then raise the back until the vertebrae fall into proper alignment. I do not want you to have such an indentation that you create a rut, as in figure 6. This means you are too flexible for this level, so go a little lower until you have a smooth groove.

Now, work at straightening your legs and maintain the smooth groove with the spine. Don't let the ischial bones turn downward because of your tight hamstrings. Keep the buttocks upward and legs as straight as you can get them, as in figure 8.

You are now executing the Standing Forward Bend from the hip socket and preserving your spinal column to move as one unit.

The ball-and-socket joint of the hip (head of the femur and acetabulum notch) is stable. It is designed for easy rotation virtually in all directions. The femoral head inserts into the acetabulum and is encapsulated there, fixed by ligaments. The pelvis adjusts to the movement of the thigh by rotating in this joint. When standing, the leg is grounded to the floor but not to the pelvis. The pelvis adjusts to the movement by rotating slightly around the head of the femur. Alignment of the pelvic girdle and grounding of the feet, knees, and thighs is essential to insure proper pelvic action and correct balance for the spine.

While it may not be apparent, the following is extremely important in all standing positions:

- The feet should be firmly grounded.
- The knees should not be locked back (hyperextended) but eased straight and lifted up toward the thighs. The buttocks should not be spread wider, but the ischial bones should be in and lifted upward to get the rotation.
- The entire front side of the torso and neck should be straight (no fold or bend).
- The smooth groove up and down the spine should have no irregularities. No vertebra(e) should be indented further or more poked out than the others. I know there will be some exceptions, but work toward balancing your unique smooth groove.

It is helpful to work with a friend and test each other, using this checklist.

As for the backward flexion of the back, when practiced

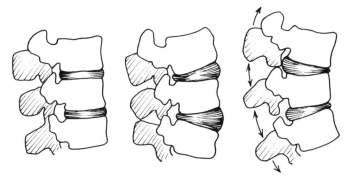

Figure 3

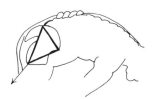

Figure 4

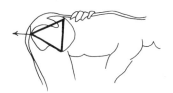

Figure 5

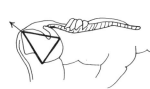

Figure 6

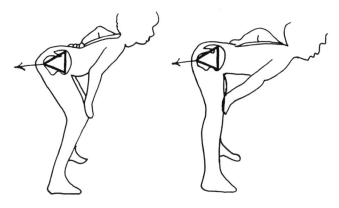

Figure 7   **Figure 8**

correctly it brings a greater blood supply to the discs and the nerves of the spinal cord. There are some important principles of backbending:

- Before arching the back, align the body and elongate the spine.
- Always tuck the tailbone downward into the body toward the pubic bone.
- Always be well-grounded in the feet and firm in the knees and pelvis throughout the entire stretch.
- Lift the spine upward, never forward, to release pressure in the lower lumbar.
- Never hold the backbending position longer than the buttocks and abdomen can stay contracted.
- Contract the abdomen with each breath. While rotating the tailbone, inhale, elongate, exhale, and contract the abdominals.
- Do not tense the neck. Keep it an extension of the spine.

The principle of the elongated and aligned spine is basic to all of my exercises, be it bending forward, backward, or laterally and must be applied until it becomes an automatic, integrated response. Notice its importance in the exercises that follow. If you have stretched properly by really aiming the top of your head and buttocks in the opposite directions, you will feel and experience the elongation in the spine.

FORWARD FLEXION: BACK ALIGNER WITH CHAIR

Props

1. A straight-backed chair against a wall or furniture.
2. A one-inch thick pole or rolled-up magazine, held together with rubber bands.

Body Placement

1. Lie down, rest your calves on top of the chair, and place your feet against the backrest to form a right angle. If the chair is too deep, stack books or something hard (not pillows) so you can push the feet into it.
2. Having your legs at a right angle will balance you on your sacrum.
3. To anchor the sacrum, lift your waist off the floor and slip under the pole. Do *not* press your spine into the pole or lift way off it. It should feel comfortable, just filling in your natural lumbar curve.
4. Review the chapter on Abdominal Muscles (section IV, chapter 4) to understand the pole and how to work the abdominals correctly.

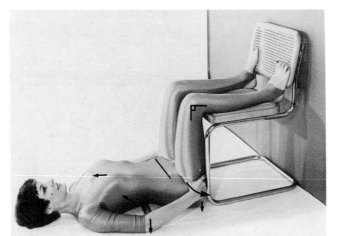

Figure 1

Technique

1. Inhale, elongating your spine up and out of the waist. While exhaling, squeeze your shoulder blades so they are tucked in and flat and rest them.
2. Place your thumbs on the thigh muscle at your frontal hip-bones. Inhale and use your thumbs and elbows for leverage to elongate, as in figure 1. While exhaling, contract your abdomen and squeeze your shoulder blades, as you dip your tailbone downward. Push with your thumbs, rotating the thigh muscle to the side and away from you. The rotating helps in the contraction of the abdominals and in squeezing the ischial bones toward each other. This aligns and balances your hips and lower back on the sacrum. Hold this balance for the count of six.
3. Repeat step 2 six times.

Variation 1

1. Repeat Technique steps 1 and 2 and once balanced at the hold position, raise your right calf and heel one inch off the chair. Hold for six counts. Repeat again, and at the same time raise your head, as in figure 2.
2. Repeat five times with each leg.

Variation 2

1. Slide away from the chair where you can get your right leg straight, as in figure 3. Keep the tailbone dipped downward and make the pole comfortable.
2. Once you have found the accurate distance for the left foot, keep the right angle and back the left foot with books. The right leg is anchored on the sacrum and the calf rests on the edge of the chair, as in figure 3.
3. Repeat Technique steps 1 and 2. Once anchored on the sacrum, use your abdominal muscles to lift the right leg away from the chair. Keep it straight and work it as close to you as you can to control a comfortable pole, as in figure 4.
4. Repeat five times and reverse, using the left leg.

Tips

1. Make sure the chair is against a wall or furniture so you won't lose your right angle.
2. Review the exercise Hamstring Stretch at Wall (section IV, chapter 2) so you can eventually do without the chair.
3. If it is still difficult for you to feel the balance on the sacrum, fold a facecloth into eighths and put it under the sacrum. Refer again to section IV, chapter 4 on Abdominal Muscles for more details.

Benefits

This exercise elongates and aligns the whole spinal column. It also balances and strengthens the pelvic girdle.

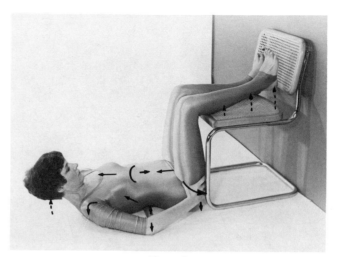

Figure 2

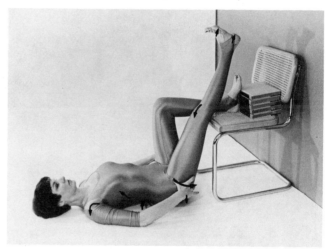

Figure 3

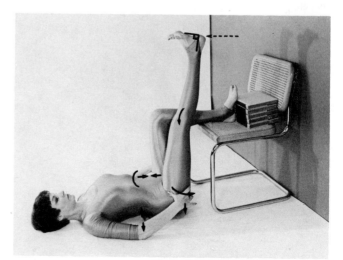

Figure 4

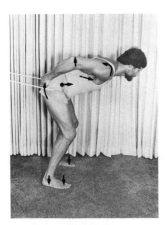

Figure 1

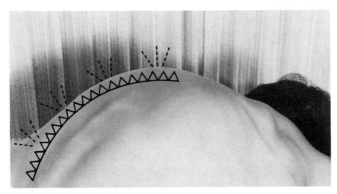

Figure 2
INCORRECT

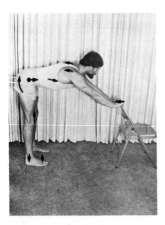

Figure 3

FORWARD FLEXION:
HANGING STANDING FORWARD BEND

Props

1. A door with doorknobs.
2. Two strong neck ties tied tightly together at both ends.
3. A chair.

Body Placement

1. Loop the ties around the doorknobs. Step through the ties, as in figure 1.
2. Place the ties under the frontal hipbone at the top of the thigh. Spread your legs three feet apart and lean into the ties. I want you to have a hanging feeling—don't worry, the doorknob won't come off.
3. Ease your knees and lift up your buttocks and ischial (sit) bones with your hands. Keep the lift as you straighten the legs—you've just found your hamstrings again!

Technique

1. While maintaining the lift in the buttocks and ischial bones with your left hand, place your right hand on the top of the chair.
2. Inhale and raise your toes, kneecaps, buttocks, and ischial bones.
3. While exhaling, take your left hand and follow up the spine for the smooth groove and work a blade squeeze.
4. If your back looks like figure 2, don't go down any further but work with your knees bent; then further raise your ischial bones. This helps to raise your back higher to get more rotation in the hips, as shown in figure 3.
5. If your back has a smooth groove with the spine recessed, as in figure 4, you can lower your straight spine to the level where the hamstrings are getting a good stretch and the lower back does not pop out or lose its alignment.
6. Stay at your own level, working the spine in and rotating your hips for three to five minutes. Take long, slow, and deep breaths. Now, isn't that a good stretch?

Variation 1

1. Notice in figure 3 the hands are put on top of the backrest of the chair after you have checked for a properly recessed spine.
2. If having your arms extended makes it difficult to rotate your hips, raise your back and bring the chair closer, while keeping the elbows bent.

Variation 2

1. The hands are on the tip of the seat, as in figure 5, only if the spine continues to be recessed.
2. If you need an in-between level, draw the chair closer to you and bend the elbows to keep your blade squeeze.

Variation 3

1. Check your recessed spine and continue to rotate your hips with the legs aligned, as in figure 6.
2. Work down with both hands on the back of the chair.

Tips

1. Make sure you do *not* hyperextend your knees. If you do, ease them and press very hard with the balls of the feet into the floor.
2. You are doing the exercise correctly if you are getting a good stretch in the hamstrings.
3. It helps to slightly pull on the chair, without moving it, to elongate your body.

Benefits

This exercise elongates and strengthens the back and makes the hip and hamstrings more flexible.

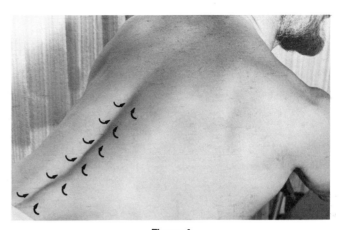

Figure 4

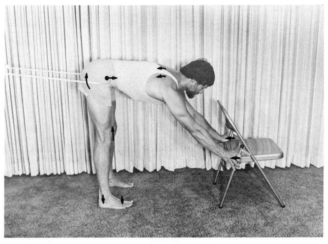

Figure 5

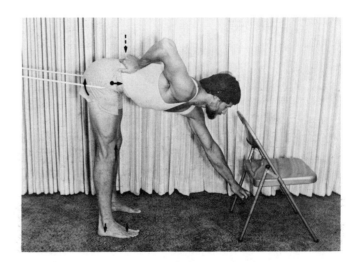

Figure 6

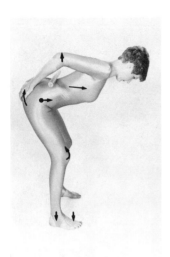

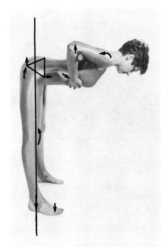

Figure 1　　　　　　　　**Figure 2**

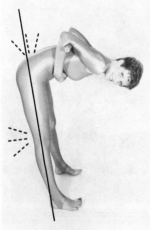

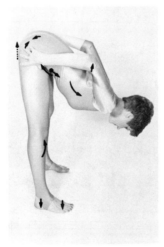

Figure 3
INCORRECT

Figure 4

FORWARD FLEXION: STANDING FORWARD BEND WITH POLE

Props

1. A one-inch wide by 2½-foot long pole.

Body Placement

1. Stand with your feet three feet apart. Put the pole across your back and at the elbows, as in figure 1.
2. While bending your knees, place the hands around the buttocks so your fingers can touch your ischial bones.
3. Lift the ischial bones as you straighten the legs and keep the pole loose, as in figure 1.

Technique

1. While inhaling, raise the toes and kneecaps as you continue to rotate your ischial bones upward. Keep your hips in line with your ankles. Do not lean your weight back beyond your heels, as in figure 3.
2. While exhaling, let go of your buttocks but keep the rotation upward. Check with your hand, to feel if you have the spine recessed into a smooth groove; then place your hands on the ribs and lift them out and forward, as in figure 2.
3. Inhale and elongate the spine, while continuing to rotate the ischial bones.
4. While exhaling, apply a blade squeeze and work your straight spine downward. Keep it away from and the elbows lightly off the pole. Don't hang onto the pole. With the thumbs between the hipbone and thighs, rotate the thigh muscle to the side and the ischial bones toward each other, as you continue to lift up the ischial bones, as in figure 4.
5. Repeat steps 1-4 five times, working yourself down. With each inhalation, increase the upward and inward rotation of the ischial bones.

Tips

1. The rotation and bend comes from the hip socket and not from the spine. The pole keeps you from bending over with the spine.
2. Make sure you align and ground your feet into the floor. This balances the hips and strengthens the legs.
3. If you hyperextend your knees, straighten them and lean into the balls of the feet.
4. If you are flexible in the hips, it is very important to concentrate on not rotating the hips by spreading the buttocks wide (ischial bones apart), which can aggravate the sacrum, hips, and lower back.

Benefits

This exercise stretches the hamstrings and strengthens the legs and back. Also, the hips become more flexible.

FORWARD FLEXION:
FORWARD BENDING HAMSTRING STRETCH

Props

None

Body Placement

1. Stand with your feet hip-width apart.
2. Place both hands so the fingers are on the ischial bones, as in figure 1. Dig in with your fingers to find the bones—they're there.

Technique

1. Inhale and bend your knees. While exhaling, rotate your shoulders back and into a blade squeeze so the elbows are shoulder-width, as in figure 2.
2. Inhale and elongate the ribs out of the waist, as you ground the feet into the floor. While exhaling, continue to rotate the ischial bones upward and keep the spine straight, as you work to straighten your legs, as in figure 3.
3. Inhale. Let go of the ischial bones and continue to recess the spine into a smooth groove. Feel your back with one hand to adjust the level of your spine so the back will be straight, as in figure 4.
4. Exhale. With the spine aligned, continue to rotate the ischiums upward, while bending forward from the hips.
5. Hold the breath out for five counts and feel a nice elongation in the spine to the top of the head. Now, stretch in the legs.
6. Repeat Technique steps 3 and 4 five more times. Come up and see how nice and straight your posture is! Feel the warmth and great stretch in the legs.

Tips

1. Make sure you do not hyperextend your knees. With the toes raised, lean forward and press the balls of the feet firmer into the floor so as not to have pressure in the back of your knees.
2. If you cannot get the spine to recess into a smooth groove, move up to where you can. When I say straighten your legs, keep your legs bent but continue to work the leverage between the legs and back.

Benefits

This exercise stretches the hamstrings and aligns and elongates the spine, while making the hips move flexibly.

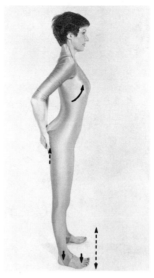

Figure 1

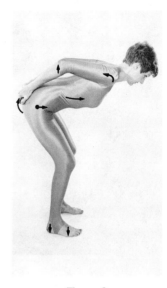

Figure 2

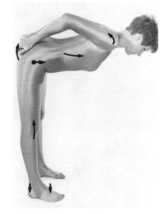

Figure 3

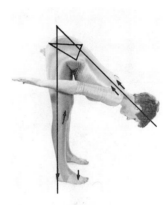

Figure 4

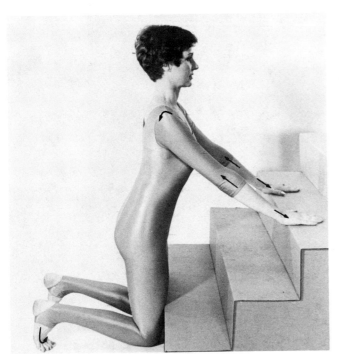

Figure 1

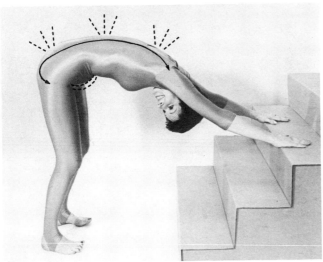

Figure 2
INCORRECT

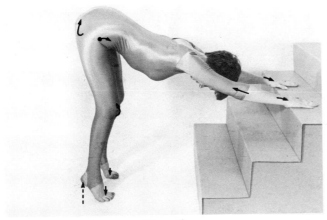

Figure 3

FORWARD FLEXION:
THE TENT

Props

1. A stairway.

Body Placement

1. Kneel up to the stairs with the knees hip-width apart and the toes curled under.
2. Place the heels of the hands shoulder-distance apart at the edge of the third step, as in figure 1.
3. Straighten the elbows. Do not rotate upward or hyperextend them. The insides of the elbows should be facing each other.
4. Move the shoulders away from your ears by drawing the outer armpits inward. Work your spine into the body, while maintaining a blade squeeze.

Technique

1. Inhale and lift the buttocks toward the ceiling. Balance up on the balls of your feet. While exhaling, completely straighten the arms. With the armpits inward, apply a push from the step to feel strength in the arms.
2. While inhaling, elongate the spine and lower your chest toward the floor. Squeeze your shoulder blades together, making a straight back, as in figure 3. Do *not* round your back, as in figure 2.
3. While exhaling, push away from the stairs and draw your head in line with your arms. The action feels as if you are being pulled and hooked up from the hips. The buttocks continues to rotate upward.
4. Inhale and keep the knees bent. Elongate the arms and spine in both directions and lengthen from the step to the tailbone.
5. While exhaling, keep the ischials rotated upward and lower your heels. Keep the arches lifted. Straighten your legs by

raising up your kneecaps toward the thighs. Do *not* move the arms or spine; they remain straight and elongated, as in figure 5. Do *not* round your back and buttocks, as in figure 4.

6. Hold the breath out as you work deeper into position.
7. Repeat Technique steps 4-6 five times.

Variation

1. Once the spine is recessed into a smooth groove and the legs are straight, work your hand down to the next step until you don't need the stairs. For each stair you lower to, step back with your feet one-foot's distance, as in figure 6.
2. Repeat Technique steps 4-6 five times.

Tips

1. If you can't rotate your ischials upward and get your back straight, keep your legs bent and up on the balls of your feet (not on the heels).
2. Keeping one hand on the step, use the other to check your spine for the smooth groove. I don't want any bumps (vertebrae protruding). Remember, it's not how you look in an exercise, it's how well you're working.
3. It is not important that your heels touch the floor. It is the alignment, strength, and stretch you feel in the back at first that counts; then, the heels may be lowered. As you become more flexible, work your hands down the steps to the floor.
4. Don't force yourself into position, let your body tell you when it is ready to go a little further.
5. As you accomplish the completed position, hold The Tent for three to five minutes for endurance.

Benefits

This exercise aligns and strengthens the arms, spine, and legs, while relieving tension in the neck and shoulder region.

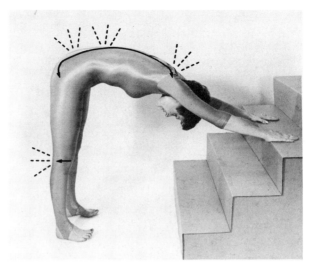

Figure 4
INCORRECT

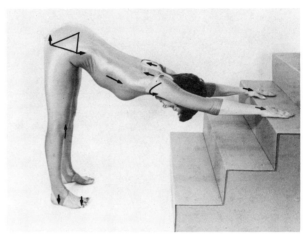

Figure 5

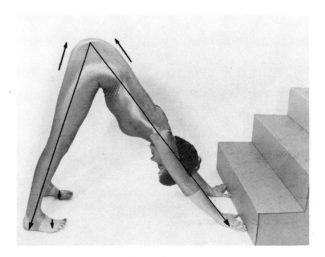

Figure 6

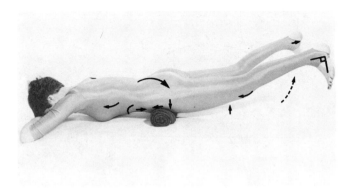

Figure 1

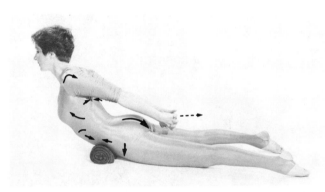

Figure 2

BACKWARD FLEXION:
THE BOAT

Props

1. A thick beach towel rolled up into a firm roll.

Body Placement

1. To raise the legs, place the roll slightly below the hipbones.
2. To raise the arms and chest, place the roll slightly above the hipbones.
3. Keep the legs hip-width apart.
4. Throughout this exercise there should *not* be any compressed pressure in the lower back. Maintain a rotation of the tailbone by tucking it downward and under as well as contracting the abdominal muscles to hold the pelvis balanced.

Technique

1. Place the roll slightly below the hipbones. Inhale and elongate the spine. While exhaling, contract the abdominals inward and tuck the tailbone down and under. Balance on the pelvic triangle.
2. Maintain the tuck and balanced pelvis on the roll. Inhale and elongate the spine out of the waist. While exhaling and still tucked, slowly raise both legs off the floor, as in figure 1. *Don't* throw the legs up and jam the back. Do it slowly. The legs won't go too high, but your back will be protected.
3. Hold for the count of five. Take in one more breath, then exhale as you work to strengthen the balance. Come down and relax.
4. Repeat Technique steps 1 and 2 three more times.

Variation 1, figure 2

1. Place the roll slightly above the hipbones. Inhale and clasp your hands behind you. Shrug your shoulders back and keep your arms straight to create a blade squeeze.
2. While exhaling, contract the abdominal muscles inward and tuck the tailbone down and under to balance on the pelvic triangle.
3. Maintain the tuck and balanced pelvis on the roll. Inhale and elongate the ribs up out of the waist. While exhaling, keep

tucked and contract the abdomen. Arch up and reach with your hands toward the feet, as in figure 2.

4. Hold for the count of five. Take in one more breath and exhale as you work to strengthen the balance. Come down and relax.

5. Repeat Variation 1, steps 1-3 three more times.

Variation 2, figure 3

1. Apply steps 1-4 from Variation 1, but open the arms out to the side and bend at the elbows, as in figure 3. You have to work harder to apply a blade squeeze. This strengthens the upper back.

2. Repeat three more times.

Variation 3, figure 4

1. Remove your roll so you can properly raise both your arms and legs at the same time.

2. Inhale and elongate. While exhaling, contract the abdomen and tuck the tailbone down and under to balance on your pelvic triangle, hipbones, and pubic bone.

3. Repeat steps 1 and 2; but on the second exhalation, first raise your arms, then your legs, as in figure 4.

4. Hold for five counts. Take one more short breath, exhale, and raise higher, working to keep the ribs off the floor. Good work! This will help you to keep your balance and elongate the lower back.

5. Repeat three more times.

Tips

1. If you cannot get or maintain the tuck and balanced pelvis when doing these exercises, move the roll up or down so you can balance on it properly. When tucking, you will be on *top* of the roll.

2. There must not be any compression (pinching) in the lower back. The lower lumbar should be elongated throughout The Boat.

Benefits

This exercise stretches and realigns the vertebrae and streamlines the legs, thighs, buttocks, and shoulders.

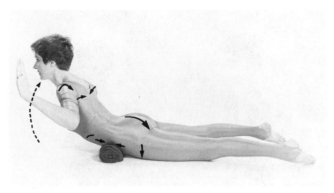

Figure 3

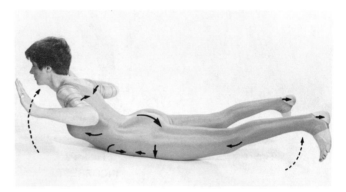

Figure 4

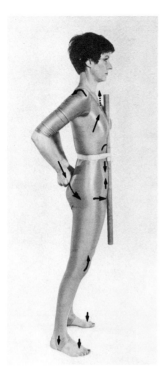

Figure 1

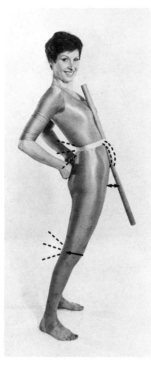

Figure 2
INCORRECT

BACKWARD FLEXION: ELONGATED BACK STRENGTHENER

Props

1. A 2½-foot pole or the attachment from a vacuum cleaner.
2. A belt with double-ring loops to slide closed.

Body Placement

1. Tie the pole *very* tightly around the waist.
2. Stand with the feet well-grounded and hip-width apart.
3. Make a fist with your hands and place them on top of your buttocks. When you squeeze the buttocks, you will have a shelf to push down on to elongate the spine.
4. Elbows are shoulder-width apart.

Technique

1. While inhaling, elongate the spine by stretching the sternum up the pole and push down with the hands on the buttocks. While exhaling, contract the abdomen and tuck the tailbone down and forward to press the pubic bone to the pole.
2. Continue repeating Technique step 1 as you tilt the spine backward, keeping the sternum and pubic bone in contact with the pole, as in figure 1. Do *not* arch your spine, as in figure 2.
3. Keep a solidly grounded support in the legs. The feet work down deeper for each elongation upward.
4. After five complete breaths, come up and relax.

Variation 1, figure 3

1. Repeat Technique steps 1-4 but place the arms out to the side, while bending at the elbows, as in figure 3. Keep elongating, while tilting back, and work to feed the spine into the body. This is a little harder because you do not have the arm support.

Variation 2, figure 4.

1. Repeat Technique steps 1-4, but place the arms along your ears shoulder-distance apart, as in figure 4.
2. As you work into your tilt, keep your feet pressing down, legs strong, and continue to reach upward with your arms. Work the arms behind your ears. It is the *lift* that is important, *not* how far you get your arms.

Tips

1. In all three Variations, the sternum is working up and to the pole. The pubic girdle is rotating to keep the pubic bone to the pole, while elongating the lumbar.
2. With each inhalation there should be a lift to elongate the spine and free it to tilt. There must not be any compression or pinching in the lower back.

Benefits

This exercise strengthens the legs, hips, and back muscles.

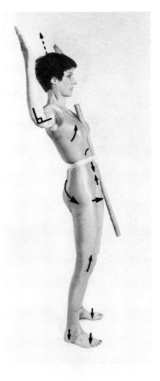

Figure 3

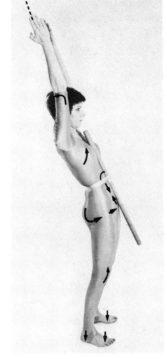

Figure 4

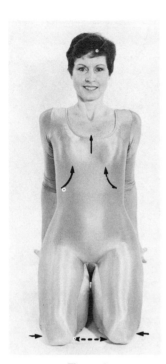

Figure 1

BACKWARD FLEXION: KNEELING VISE

Props

1. Optional, two cans of tunafish.

Body Placement

1. Sit on the floor with the legs bent at the knees, feet beside the buttocks, and hands behind the toes.
2. When kneeling, we tend to roll out to the outside of our knees. This pulls on the ligaments. To bend with the knees centered, place the knees hip-distance apart and slide the knee joint within the skin. Keep this squeeze in the thighs and buttocks, as in figure 1.
3. Take five breaths and work deeper into your position. Come out and relax.

Technique

1. Inhale and elongate the spine by lifting the ribs up and out of the waist. Lean back on the fingertips.
2. While exhaling, rotate the tailbone under to lead the pubic bone forward and contract the abdominals, as in figure 3. Do not let the knees spread apart and back arch, as in figure 2. This puts pressure in the lower back—Ouch!
3. Hold the breath out for five counts.
4. Repeat steps 1-3 five times to further tighten the vise (rotation of the pelvis). Come out and relax. You thought this would be easy?

Variation 1, figure 4, Elbows

1. Repeat Technique steps 1-3. Working from the fingertips to down on your elbows, contract the abdominals and maintain all the proper alignment.
2. Keep rotating the pubic bone forward to line up with the thighs, hipbones, and ribs, as in figure 4.

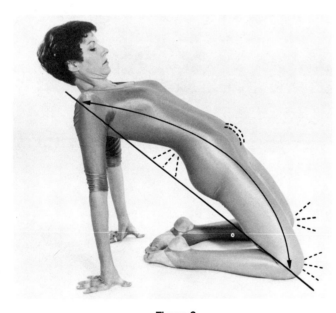

Figure 2
INCORRECT

Variation 2, figure 5, Supine

1. Repeat Technique steps 1-3 and work from the elbows to lying down on the floor, as in figure 5.
2. If the knees spring up off the floor, place one or two of the tuna cans under your sacrum to elevate and rotate the pelvic girdle properly. Don't let the lower back arch; keep it elongated by breathing the ribs in and down from the sides, *not* upward.
3. Take five breaths and work deeper into your position. Come out and relax.

Tips

1. I recommend you review the Kneeling Thigh Tilt (section IV, chapter 2) before doing the Kneeling Vise. It will give you a good foundation from which to work.
2. If the pelvic rotation is difficult for you to acquire, tie a pole around your waist, as in the Kneeling Thigh Tilt, to act as a reminder when you lose the control.
3. If your knees spread out wider than your hips, you should not lower yourself from that point. Tie a belt around your thighs to keep the knee in, but don't push into the belt. Keep it loose.

Benefits

This exercise stretches the thighs and tones the legs and buttocks, while stimulating the abdominal organs and pelvic region.

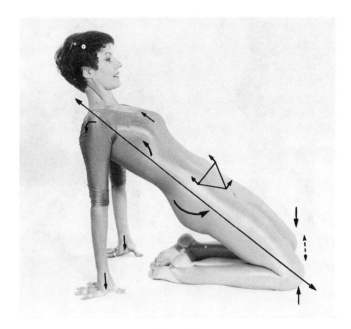

Figure 3

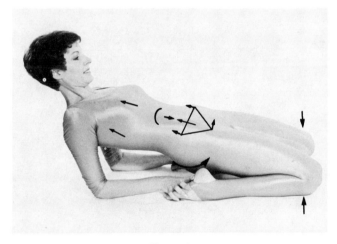

Figure 4

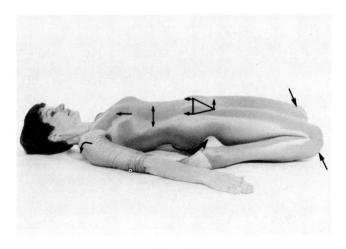

Figure 5

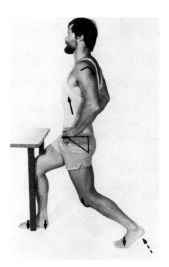

Figure 1

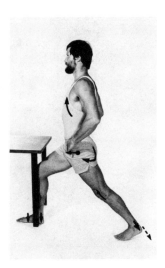

Figure 2

BACKWARD FLEXION: SIDE FACING PLUNGE

Props

1. An outside corner.

Body Placement

1. Stand with your feet four feet apart. Rotate the legs and pivot on the right heel, turning the foot out and lining up the ankle with the corner. Rotate and pivot, turning the left foot in, as in figure 1.
2. Place your hands on your hips to steer and monitor a vertical pelvic triangle. While bending the right knee, rotate the left hip to face the corner. Make sure both hips are level and even, as in figure 1. If not, bring the feet closer together.

Technique

1. Inhale, and press the left foot down, while lifting the toes, foot arch, and kneecap. Elongate the spine up out of the waist.
2. While exhaling, bend the left knee to square off the left hip. Keep your left hip even with the right one.
3. Inhale and elongate. While exhaling, rotate the tailbone downward to draw the pubic bone forward to make the pelvic triangle completely vertical and face evenly with the corner.
4. Inhale and elongate the spine. While exhaling, contract the abdoninals, apply a blade squeeze, and draw the shoulders to line up with the hips, as in figure 1. Do *not* lean forward with the hips ahead of the pubic bone, as in figure 3.
5. Inhale and maintain the elongation and alignment of the spine. While exhaling, contract the abdominals and keep the left hip forward. As you raise up the left kneecap, straighten out the left leg and lower the heel, as in figure 2. If you can do this, repeat Technique steps 1-5 with the legs further apart so you can accomplish a right angle, as in figure 4. Looks easy, doesn't it?
6. Repeat Technique steps 3-5 six times, working in an aligned, balanced position.
7. Come out and repeat with the left leg.

Breathing Rhythm

1. Inhale means to elongate and reinforce the balance of the body by grounding your position.
2. Exhale means to contract the abdominals, secure the vertical pelvic triangle, and work into the position *only* if the body is open and accepts the advancement.
3. Hold means you hold out the exhalation and hold the balance in the new position so it can be adjusted and accepted.
4. Repeat the cycle.
5. When you have had enough, come out of it and repeat on the other side.

Variation 1 (not shown)

1. Raise your arms, stretching up overhead, *only* if the left heel is on the floor, the right thigh and calf form a right angle, and, most importantly, the pelvic triangle is completely vertical.
2. Lift from your ribs, not from your shoulders. The neck remains centered and relaxed with the elbows straight and arms up by the ears.

Tips

1. In the beginning it helps to hold onto the corner for balance. You can then put more strength and alignment into the exercise.
2. Tying the pole to you can be a tremendous aid in maintaining the alignment.
3. It is also helpful to do this in front of a mirror. View yourself from the front and side.

Benefits

This exercise builds stamina in the legs and hip region, while toning up the ankles and knees.

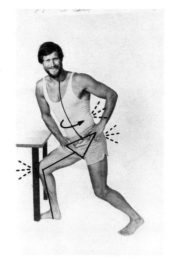

Figure 3
INCORRECT

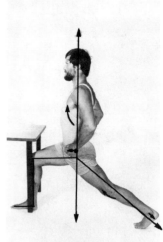

Figure 4

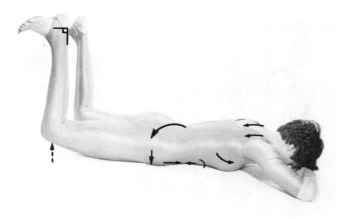

Figure 1

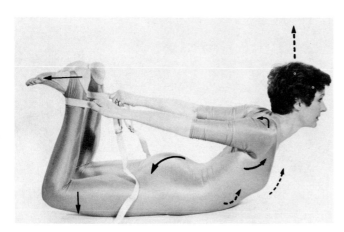

Figure 2
INCORRECT

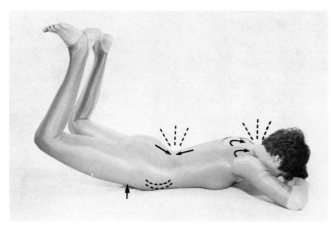

Figure 3

BACKWARD FLEXION:
THE BOW

Props

1. Optional, two belts.

Body Placement

1. Lie on your stomach with your hands under your fore-head. Shrug your shoulders down away from your ears.
2. Knees are hip-distance apart. Your legs remain parallel with the feet flexed so the soles face the ceiling.
3. Rotate the tailbone down and under, while contracting the abdominals so the navel lifts inward. The pubic bone and frontal hipbones are the foundation of this exercise.

Technique

1. Inhale and elongate the spine and ribs up out of your waist.
2. While exhaling, rotate the tailbone down and under and contract the abdominals to anchor the pelvic triangle foundation.
3. Inhale and elongate without drawing the shoulders up; they should remain rotated in a blade squeeze. While exhaling, stabilize the foundation and raise the thighs off the floor, as in figure 1. They will not come up too high, but notice the strength and control in the lower back. Compare the extension in the lower back and thigh in figures 1 and 2.
4. Hold for a count of five. Repeat one more breath to reinforce the stabilization of your foundation.
5. Come down and rest. Did you think that would be easy?

Variation 1, figure 3, Chest Up with Belt

1. If you find it difficult to grab your ankles, looping two belts at the ankles will give you the length you need. Hold onto the belts with your shoulders shrugged back and down, away from the ears, into a tight shoulder blade squeeze, as in figure 3.
2. Inhale and elongate the spine forward and upward. While exhaling, stabilize your foundation by contracting the abdominals and ribs. Keep the thighs on the floor and the arms taut. This creates a bowstring effect.
3. Inhale and increase the elongation. While exhaling, press the ankles into the belt and stabilize your foundation and balance by working the ribs off the floor, as in figure 3.
4. Hold for five counts. Use this breathing pattern for two more rounds. Continuously lift the chest higher. Come down and rest.

Variation 2, figure 4, Chest Up without Belt

1. Repeat Variation 1, steps 2-4, but grab your ankles with your hands, as in figure 4.
2. Don't push the abdominals into the floor, but contract them inward. The neck extends up out of the shoulders but is also relaxed. Keep the bow effect between the shoulders and feet, as you slowly raise your chest and ribs off the floor. Stay on the pubic bone; don't lift off it.

Variation 3, figure 6, Both Ends Up

1. Raise both ends at the same time; but before you do, compare figures 5 and 6. Don't lose your pelvic foundation as in figure 5. Here, the pubic bone is off the floor, compressing the lower lumbar, which can in time create damage to the vertebrae from incorrect bending.
2. Holding onto the ankles, inhale and elongate the spine forward and upward.
3. While exhaling, rotate the tailbone and contract the abdominals and ribs to stabilize your pelvic foundation. Keep the pubic bone rooted to the floor.
4. Inhale and increase the elongation and tautness in the arms and shoulders.
5. While exhaling, keep the stabilized foundation and reach to the ceiling with the top of the head and the soles of the feet, as in figure 6.
6. Hold for five counts. Use this breathing pattern for two more rounds, continuously reaching higher. Come down and relax. Great, you did it!

Tips

1. There should be no need to round your back for relief if the exercise is done correctly. It is a good way to monitor the quality of your work. Each of my exercises is complete in itself and needs no relief if done properly.
2. Do *not* swing yourself up with momentum; that is *not* working from control.
3. Keep your legs parallel. I know they want to swing out; but work more from the hips and tighten the pelvic foundation. To get the proper action, tie a belt around the thighs. Then work independent of it.

Benefits

This exercise greatly strengthens and develops the entire spine, while freeing the lumbar area. It opens the chest and reduces the hips and buttocks, while stretching the groin.

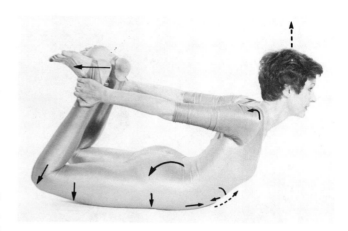

Figure 4

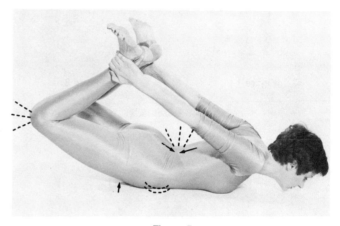

**Figure 5
INCORRECT**

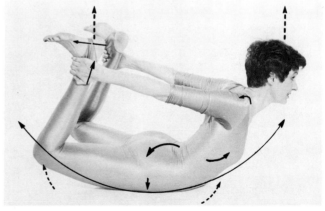

Figure 6

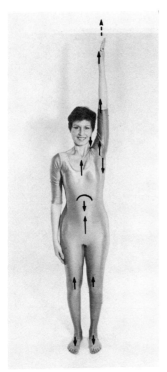

Figure 1

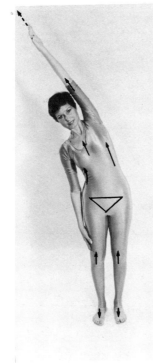

Figure 2

LATERAL STRETCH AND TWIST: LATERAL STRETCH

Props
None

Body Placement
1. Stand with the feet a comfortable distance apart. The feet should stay grounded (well-rooted) into the floor.
2. Raise up the kneecaps with the legs straight, not hyperextended.
3. The pelvic triangle is to remain vertical at all times, which means keep the pubic bone forward in line with the hipbones.
4. Shoulders remain down, away from the ears, with a squaring off of the shoulders into a blade squeeze.
5. To free the shoulder joint, first bend the elbows. Then work the stretch from the ribs as the arm straightens.

Technique
1. While inhaling, ground the feet and raise up the kneecaps. Straighten the legs as you elongate the spine.
2. While exhaling, tuck the tailbone down and through to draw the pubic bone forward to line up with the hipbones and pelvic triangle. At the same time, contract the abdominals.
3. Inhale and elongate. Raise up the left arm along the ear, as in figure 1. While exhaling, stabilize the pelvic triangle, enfore a blade squeeze, and contract the abdominals. While reaching upward, tilt to the side and continue to stretch diagonally, as in figure 2.
4. To tilt, reach *upward*. This is not a side bend where you fold in at the waist, as in figures 3a and 4a.

5. Extend out of the tilt a little. While inhaling, press the left foot deeper into the floor and elongate from the hips all the way to the fingertips. There is room for stretch at each joint as indicated by the dotted arrows, as in figure 3b.

6. While exhaling, stabilize the pelvic triangle, contract the abdominals, maintain the elongation, and further tilt diagonally, as in figures 3b and 4b. Note the alignment of both the front and side views.

7. Hold for five counts. Repeat one more cycle. Raise up the arm and lower to the side. (Feel a little taller on one side?) Repeat with the left arm and complete four times on each side.

Tips

1. Keep the shoulders squared off away from the ears. It is helpful in freeing the shoulder joint to bend the elbow a little on the first tilt to insure a tighter blade squeeze. Refer to the Blade Squeeze with Pole (section IV, chapter 6) for more details. Straighten the arm and stretch from the ribs. The reach does *not* come from the neck.

2. As you tilt the legs and feet, continue to move downward to ground yourself.

3. Study closely figures 2 and 3b and practice in front of a mirror to check your alignment. Wearing the pole tied to you greatly helps in keeping you aligned.

Benefits

This exercise elongates and strengthens the spinal column and slims the waist and midriff bulge.

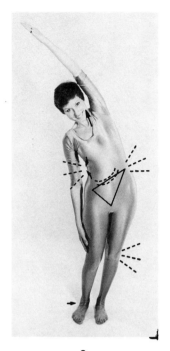
a
INCORRECT

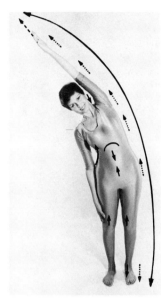
b

Figure 3

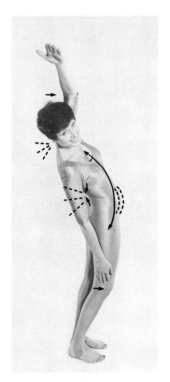
a
INCORRECT

b

Figure 4

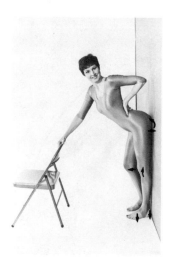

Figure 1

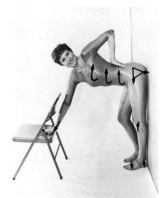

Figure 2

LATERAL STRETCH AND TWIST: STANDING BENT LEG TWIST

Props

1. A chair.
2. A wall.

Body Placement

1. Stand with your heels hip-distance apart at or slightly away from the wall, depending on the size of your calves.
2. Place your right hand on top of the backrest of the chair and bend the elbow. The left arm is bent back so the hand can feel for the smooth groove of the recessed spine, as in figure 1.
3. Bend the right knee and *press* ("screw") the two ischial bones to the wall. They should be continuously screwed with equal pressure to the wall.
4. The hand placement on the chair depends on your flexibility. Keep feeling your back for the smooth groove. If you have or get a deep gully, you should move down to where you can work a smooth groove, recessing the vertebrae all the way up the spine. Study the hand and spine positions of figures 1-4.

Technique

1. Inhale and elongate the spine with the two ischial bones as the base of the twist. They should be evenly secured into the wall. The extension follows deep into the spine and comes out the top of the head.
2. While exhaling, rotate the right shoulder back and down. Pull the elbow behind you and apply a deeper blade squeeze.
3. Inhale and continue to elongate in *both* directions, from your head to your ischial bones, as well as having your feet firmly grounded into the floor.

4. Exhale. From the downward action in the legs, rotate the ischial bones up the wall. Start the twist from the base of the hips and screwed ischial bones into a smooth, straight grooved spine—feel it with your hand. Keeping your chin in line with the sternum makes the neck act as a continuation of the twist.

5. Partly ease out of the twist and repeat Technique steps 1-5 four times. Come out of the twist slowly, unscrewing yourself, and repeat on the other side.

Tips

1. In executing a twist properly, don't turn and twist from your weakest or most flexible areas. The spine must be grounded and stabilized by screwing the two ischial bones into the wall. Think of a spiral staircase on its side, the vertebrae being the steps encircling the spinal column.

2. You *must* maintain the elongation before each rotation to employ the proper distance in the discs to insure a healthy rotation of the vertebrae. Elongation is a big key.

3. I know the bent-leg ischial bone wants to come off the wall, but don't let it. Keep it "screwed," pressing into the wall; but you may lower it to aid in the twist.

4. While twisting, the left and right side of the waist and rib cage should be equally long, straight, and parallel to each other.

Benefits

This exercise realigns the vertebrae and relieves tension in the whole spine, while massaging the internal organs. It is also a good stretch for the hamstrings.

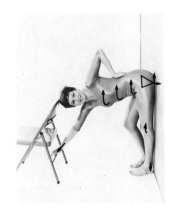

Figure 3

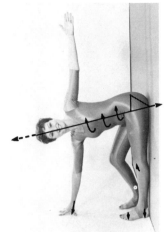

Figure 4

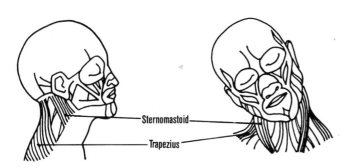

Sternomastoid

Trapezius

6. Chest, Shoulder Girdle, Neck, and Eyes

Remember the four curves of the back from the previous chapter? The neck is one of these called the cervical, although it is often not acknowledged as part of the spine. When alignment is lost in one of the other curves, the neck is pushed out of balance and tension or pain occurs.

There is more to the cervical column then you might expect. You can see that the normal neck has a curve on the back side. A straight neck is not desirable because it does not bear weight and shock well. What we can't see is that it functions as a canal for the arteries and spinal cord. The bones and the nerves of the neck are very closely connected. Anytime you move your neck, you're not just moving bones and ligaments; you're also moving nerves and blood vessels.

The neck muscle most vulnerable to strain is the trapezius. It runs from the base of the skull down the back of the neck, where it fans out to the shoulder blades and spine. The sternomastoid muscle supports the neck to the sides and front, just as the trapezius does to the sides and back.

There are many causes that contribute to neck strain and headaches, such as wearing high heels, slumping over a desk or looking into a computer, carrying a shoulder bag or suitcase, being scrunched up to a telephone receiver, bad posture, and mental stress. When any of these occur for a continued length of time, the more likely the muscles will knot, which puts a pressure on the blood flow. The body reacts in a pain-spasm-pain cycle. This is all the more reason for the corrective elongating exercises that are in this chapter.

To test your neck mobility and alignment, sit on the edge of your chair and put your hands on the back of your neck, interlocking your fingers. While rounding your back, drop your chin toward your chest. You will be feeling the action at vertebrae C1-C6. Bend the head forward, backward, and from side to side, feeling which vertebra sticks out the most. See how the apex of movement shifts, showing you your area of greatest wear and strain.

Now, with your fingers still on the neck, sit up straight and balance on your ischial bones. As you properly align your posture, with your chest up and open and shoulders rolled back and down, balance your head above your shoulders. Bend your head forward, backward, and from side to side again, as if a string is gently pulling upward from the top of your head. Notice the freedom in the action and the ease in the muscles as you rotate your neck—you are maintaining the four natural curves of the whole spinal column.

The shoulder girdle and the thoracic area of the spine are responsible for the balance of the neck. If you look like you are carrying the world on your shoulders, you will notice your head fall forward and tightness in your neck and/or shoulders.

The shoulder girdle is strong and reliable and one of the largest joints of the body; but it is not a weight-bearing mechanism. Because of this and its unique design and mobility, the shoulder girdle has a wide range of motion. Since it possesses mobility in many directions, many more muscles are required to move and support it than other joints. As a result, the area of the shoulders is jam-packed with muscles and tendons that crisscross, intertwine, overlap, and interact.

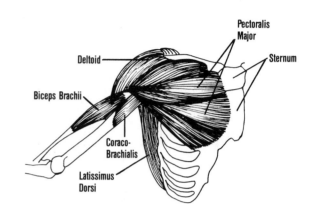

These muscle groups share many functions: lifting of the ribs, extension of the sternum in the front, balance of the shoulders on top, and alignment of the shoulder blades in the back. The muscles all act in concert, some coming into play more strenuously than others, depending on the precise direction of the movement. If the movement required of the shoulder girdle, from a particular sport or activity, is out of alignment with the rest of the body, it puts strain on the neck and/or lower back.

For example, when I read about or see exercises done where the instructions say to keep the back flat, "pressed to the floor," as in Leg Raises, I shudder to think, and feel, what is happening to the neck. When you change the natural curvature of the lumbar vertebrae, you make the neck arch backward and vice versa. This shows the uselessness of fragmentary work. Read the chapter on Abdominal Muscles (section IV, chapter 4) for more details. It's absolutely necessary to regard your body as a totality and bring your unique body into attaining proper alignment.

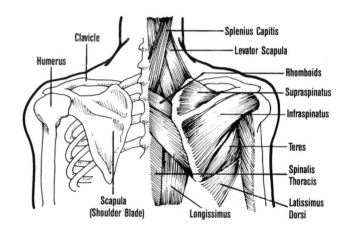

It's a tricky engineering job for the body to hold itself upright. It's like balancing a watermelon on a broomstick by the support system of large elastic bands (muscles). Imbalances, such as a concave chest, tension-prone neck, and weak, unresponsive arms can lead to a stiff shoulder girdle. Continued bad posture weakens the upper body and taxes the lower body by making it work harder to carry and balance a full torso. Those stiff and immovable joints and muscles cause discomfort and pain. This is why I have emphasized the Blade Squeeze and illustrated it with directive arrows that show both a downward and an inward stroke. Most people will try to hunch their shoulders upward in an attempt to squeeze their blades. Instead, the neck gets squeezed. These people need the enforcement of the directive arrows in the exercises. For women to put the Blade Squeeze action in the right place, think of trying to unsnap the bra in the back with no hands. There is the right spot on which to concentrate.

As your shoulder girdle comes into alignment, there is no need to squeeze the shoulder blades. You can now work at further opening the chest by keeping the downward stroke and adding the action of broadening your flat shoulder blades. For you more experienced students, make the notation by drawing over the inward arrows and reverse the direction.

When you work on your shoulder and neck regions, observe the body as a whole (totality). Work with the following exercises to attain your unique alignment.

CHEST OPENER

Props

1. A 2½-foot long pole or vacuum attachment.
2. A belt.
3. A mirror.

Body Placement

1. Stand in a straight, aligned posture with your feet grounded and the pelvic triangle maintaining a vertical position for each of the Chest Opener exercises.

Technique

1. Inhale, elongate the ribs out of the waist, and extend the sternum up and forward.
2. While exhaling, align the pelvic triangle and contract the abdominals. Rotate your shoulders back and downward, creating a blade squeeze.
3. Hold the breath out for the count of five, while working the upper thoracic spine deeper into the body and opening the chest.
4. Repeat the cycle five times.

Variation 1, figure 1a, with Pole

1. Place the pole at the bend of the elbow, as in figure 1a.
2. Repeat Technique steps 1-4, while working the spine and elbows away from the pole.

Variation 2, figure 1b, with Belt

1. Clasp onto a belt with your hands hip-distance apart. Note that the palms of the hands are toward the buttocks, as in figure 1b.
2. Repeat Technique steps 1-4, while working your arms straight down and away from the body with the belt. As you become more open you can inch your hands in closer together.
3. Do not sacrifice the elongation and extended sternum by trying to raise the belt too high. I bet you're standing a little straighter now.

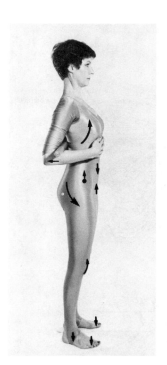
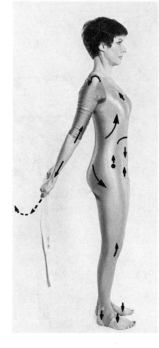

a   b

Figure 1

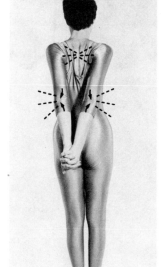
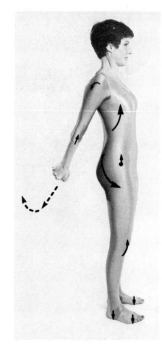

a   b

INCORRECT

Figure 2

Variation 3, figure 2, with Hands Clasped

1. Clasp your hands together. While shrugging your shoulders down away from your ears, execute a blade squeeze to straighten the arms, as in figure 2b, *not* hyperextended, as in figure 2a. If so, ease your arms to get them straight. The work is in the shoulders, not in the elbows. Read section IV, chapter 7.
2. Repeat Technique steps 1-4, while working to open the chest and lift the arms higher.

Variation 4, figure 3, Blade Squeeze

1. Outstretch your arms to the side at shoulder level.
2. Repeat Technique steps 1-4, while executing a blade squeeze down away from the ears and squeezing the lower edges of the blades without any props, as in figure 3a, *not* as in figure 3b, all hunched up near the shoulders.
3. Inhale and lengthen your outstretched arms. While exhaling, draw the arms in and execute a low blade squeeze. Do *not* throw your arms back; they should stay in line with the shoulders.

Variation 5, figure 4, Raising Arms Overhead

1. Applying Technique steps 1-4, maintain the lower blade squeeze as you raise the arms up along the ears, as in figure 4b, *not* as in figure 4a, all hunched up. To strengthen the squared-off shoulders, roll the outer edge of your armpit in toward the body. When you get to this level, work to broaden the flat shoulder blades downward and extend the sternum upward.

Tips

1. I encourage beginners to extend or thrust the ribs and chest upward and forward.
2. Experienced students with a good blade squeeze and open chest should not thrust the ribs out forward. I advise them to breathe into the back of the ribs and contract the ribs in from the sides on the exhale. This draws the work deeper into the upper thoracic area and maintains proper body alignment.
3. Don't pull or strain at the props; they are aids to help you work more freely in your body.

Benefits

This exercise increases lung capacity, eases tension in the shoulders and upper back, and remedies dowager's hump.

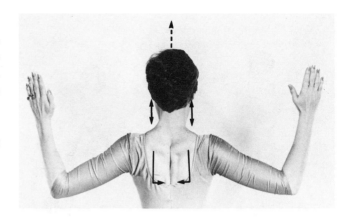

a

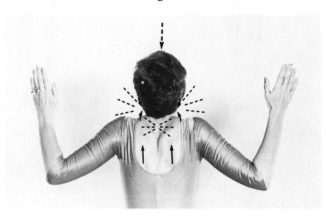

b
INCORRECT
Figure 3

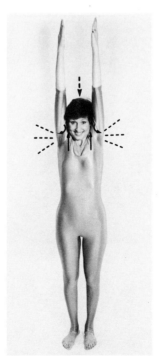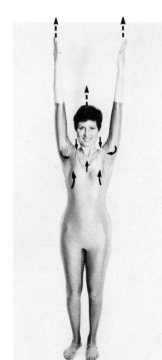

a   b
INCORRECT

Figure 4

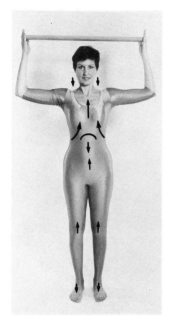

Figure 1

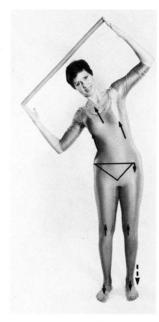

Figure 2

BLADE SQUEEZE WITH POLE

Props

1. A 2½-foot long pole or vacuum attachment.
2. A set of three-pound weights.
3. A mirror.

Body Placement

1. Stand with your feet parallel and a comfortable distance apart, while maintaining proper body alignment.
2. Clasp the pole with your palms facing each other. Keep the pole centered over your head and your elbows bent at shoulder level. Keeping your shoulders down away from your ears, execute a blade squeeze, as in figure 1.

Technique

1. Inhale and elongate the spine from the sternum, *not* from the shoulders.
2. While exhaling, rotate the pelvic triangle vertically and contract the abdominals. Keep your shoulders down and arms slightly behind your ears as you tilt to the side, as in figure 2.
3. Hold for the count of five, while aligning the balance. Come back up from the tilt.
4. Repeat the cycle four more times.

Variation 1, Tilt with Pole

1. Apply Technique steps 1-4, while tilting to the side, as in figure 2. Do *not* arch the back or fold to the side at the waist. Remember to ground yourself with your opposite foot when you tilt.
2. Keep an elongated tilt with the pole. Elbows, shoulders, and hips should be in one line. Turn sideways to check your alignment in the mirror

Variation 2, Lifting Weights

1. Slide pole through the set of weights and rest on top of shoulders, as in figure 3.
2. Apply Technique steps 1-3, while raising the weights up over your head, as in figure 4. As you slowly raise up the weights, the lower you should work the shoulder blades. This aligns and strengthens your lift.
3. Repeat the cycle five more times.

Tips

1. Review the Lateral Stretch (section IV, chapter 5) to insure that you understand the side alignment as well as the front and back ones.
2. Keep the pelvic triangle vertical at all times. The centering control comes from the contracted abdominals
3. You may widen the blade space *only* if your thoracic posture is aligned.

Benefits

This exercise aids in bursitis, releases tension in the shoulders, and slims midriff bulge.

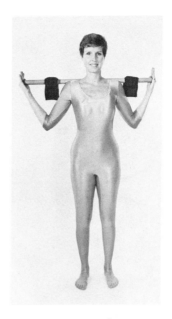

Figure 3

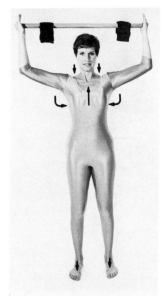

Figure 4

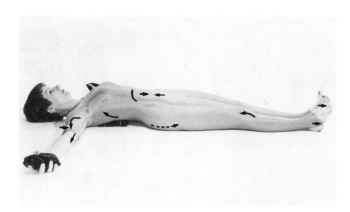

Figure 1

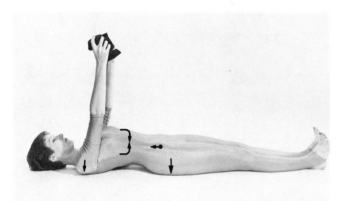

Figure 2

SUPINE BLADE SQUEEZE

Props

1. A set of two- or three-pound weights.
2. A facecloth folded in half, rolled up tightly, and held together with rubber bands.

Body Placement

1. Lie down and place the rolled facecloth lengthwise under your spine between the lower edges of the shoulder blades.
2. Outstretch the arms at shoulder level and grab the whole weight in the palms of the hands, as in figure 1.

Technique

1. Inhale and elongate the spine by extending the sternum.
2. While exhaling, rotate the shoulders down and execute a blade squeeze around the facecloth. You should hardly know it is there.

Variation 1, Lifting Weights

1. Apply Technique steps 1 and 2. Inhale and extend the sternum. Exhale and squeeze the blades downward and inward. Contract the ribs and abdominals. Straighten your arms and slowly lift the weight by squeezing the blades more to engulf the facecloth, as in figure 2. Hold the breath out with your arms up at shoulder-width.
2. While inhaling, extend the sternum and ground your flat shoulder blades. While exhaling, slowly lower your arms and keep the facecloth engulfed.
3. Repeat five times.

Variation 2, Arms Overhead

1. With your arms at your sides, apply Technique steps 1 and 2. Inhale and extend the sternum. While exhaling, blade squeeze

and contract the abdominals. Raise your arms in line with your face, shoulder-width apart, as in figure 3.

2. While inhaling, extend the sternum and ground your flat shoulder blades. While exhaling, rotate the outer edges of your armpits in toward the body and turn the arms so the palms aim overhead, not at each other.

3. Now, lower the arms overhead. Do *not* bend the elbows so the hands touch the floor. Go lower only as far as you can keep the facecloth engulfed and your back from arching. (Remember the pole!) Keep your armpits turned inward without popping the ribs up. When coming up, exhale and contract the abdominals and ribs as tight as you can.

4. The shoulder joint will free in time. *Don't* force. Breathe into this position, repeating Technique steps 1 and 2. After five breaths, come up.

5. Repeat four more times.

Tips

1. For beginners, I can't say enough about the importance of squeezing the lower shoulder blades to align the shoulder girdle and free the shoulder joints.

2. When it is too easy to lower the arms flat on the floor overhead, start breathing into the back of the ribs and contract the ribs in from the sides on exhalation. This further works and aligns the upper body. When you feel ready, you may use three-pound weights—but no more!

Benefits

This exercise frees the rotation of the shoulder joint and opens the chest.

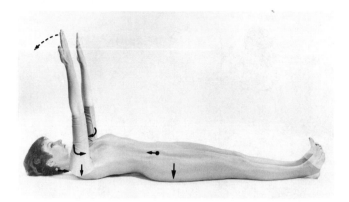

Figure 3

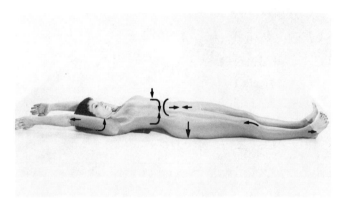

Figure 4

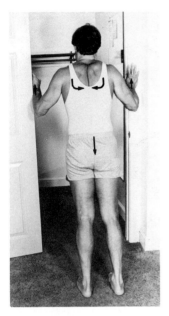

Figure 1

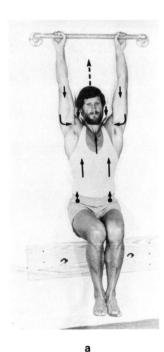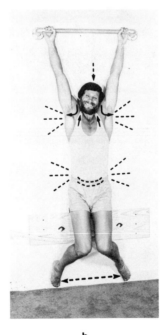

a   b

                INCORRECT

Figure 2

SHOULDER OPENER

Props

1. A door and doorway or an inside corner at a wall.
2. A chin bar.
3. A chair.
4. A sink or counter top.

Body Placement

1. In all of the Shoulder Openers, your spine is elongated and aligned with the shoulders down and back away from the ears and you execute a blade squeeze.
2. In each position maintain a balanced and aligned pelvic girdle. Do *not* let your back arch.

Technique

1. While inhaling, elongate the spine by extending the sternum up and forward and rotate the shoulders back and down.
2. While exhaling, tuck the tailbone down and under and contract the abdominals. Execute a deep blade squeeze as you lift the chest up and open. Align the shoulder girdle.
3. Hold the breath out and this position for the count of five.
4. Repeat five more times.

Variation 1, figure 1, At Doorway or Corner

1. Stand in front of a doorway with your hands at rib level and elbows behind the ribs, as in figure 1.
2. Standing in perfect posture, repeat Technique steps 1-4. While pushing the doorway with your hands, lean forward to open your chest and free the shoulder joint. Keep in line with your wrist. *Don't* just hang forward—*push* to align the chest and shoulders. If you are at a corner, push your hands sideways at chest level.

Variation 2, figure 2, Hanging

1. Grab hold of the chin bar or top of the door. Let yourself hang incorrectly, as in figure 2b. Totally let go. You will notice your armpits are opened, neck is sunken into your shoulders, and shoulder joints are weak.
2. To align yourself and hang correctly, repeat Technique steps 1-3 with the feet on the floor and legs bent (sort of sitting). Keep your arms absolutely straight and the outer edge of the armpits rotating inward. Elongate the spine up through the body by working the shoulders downward, as in figure 2a. When you feel your shoulders and arms are strong, lift up your legs to form a right angle and elongate. You will feel like a snake lifting out of its skin. Hold for three counts, drop down a little, and lift up again.
3. Repeat three more times.

Variation 3, figure 3, Praying

1. Kneel in front of a chair where you will work to lower your head, chest, and blades to align up with your hips, as in figure 3. Your elbows are shoulder-width apart. Place the palms of your hands on your arms and look up at the back of the chair. As you work to elongate and open in the shoulders, the head will come in line. *Don't* force. If you are jammed, move your arms away from your head.

2. Repeat Technique steps 1-3, while *pressing* down with your elbows onto the edge of the chair and square off the shoulders. Keep pressing to open and strengthen the shoulder joint, as the spine is able to align and lower. *Don't* just let the elbows roll out and hang down and *don't* lead with your ribs and head. The elbows want to slide out inside the skin. Stay on top of the flat area and keep your elbow joints toward each other but still shoulder-distance apart. *Press* the elbows in and down, elongate the spine in two directions, apply a deeper blade squeeze, and contract the abdominals and ribs. There should not be any tension in the neck or lower back. Let the head follow in alignment as you open in the shoulders.

3. Stay in this position for five breaths. Come up and relax.

Variation 4, figure 4, At the Sink

1. Stand in front of your sink with your elbows barely off the edge (so that little bone won't hurt). Hold onto the sink with your hands. Press the elbows down to square off the shoulders and bring up the head to look at the hands.

2. Repeat Technique steps 1-3. While keeping the shoulders squared off, work to deepen your blade squeeze and elongate the spine. Think of or let someone *pull* your hips as you hold on tight with your hands. As your partner pulls you, align your body with a deeper blade squeeze, a recessed spine, and strongly contracted abdominals. The elbows, shoulders, ribs, and hips are in a straight horizontal line. The neck is relaxed with the ears in line with the arms, and the ankles are under the hips, as in figure 4. When you are being pulled, work a stronger elongation. Draw the top of your head toward the sink, as if pulling the spine out of its skin.

3. Continue resisting for five breaths. Come up and relax. Feel a little taller?

Tips

1. Depending on your height, the chair or sink may not be appropriate. The rule to go by is to have them at your hip level.

2. For Hanging (Variation 2, figure 2), the chin bar should be only at the height where you need to get up on your toes to grab it. If it is too high, step up on something. *Don't* jump up to grab it and *don't* arch the back.

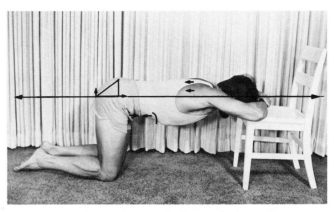

Figure 3

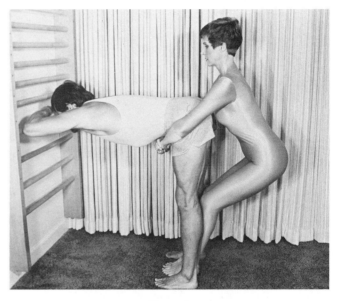

Figure 4

Benefits

This exercise stretches and strengthens the shoulder joint, upper back, and pectoral muscles. It also reduces bursitis and arthritic pain.

TWISTING WITH A CHAIR

Props

1. A chair with a hard seat.

Body Placement

1. The spine must be grounded on the two ischial bones; that is, you sit straight down into the chair. Review the Daily Living Habits (section V, chapter 3) for the corrective sitting positions.
2. Think of a spiral staircase with the pelvic girdle as its base, as in figure 1a. The stairs are the vertebrae that encircle the spinal column, and the spaces between the stairs are the discs that need to be elongated to insure a healthy rotation (twist).
3. After you have reviewed the corrective sitting posture, sit backward on the edge of the chair with both knees to the left of the chair. Place your hands on top of the corners of the backrest, as in figure 1b.
4. I know it's hard to fit both ischial bones on the seat; but if you lift up the right knee by getting up on the toes (Look closely at figure 1b.), you can adjust yourself to fit or try a different chair.

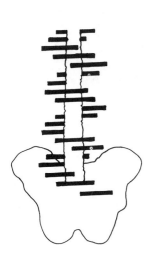
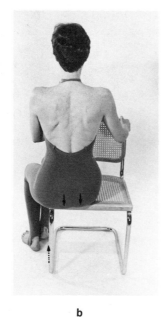

a   b

Figure 1

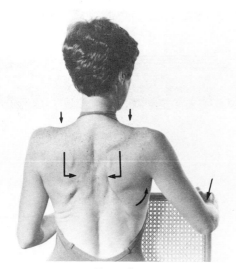

Figure 2

Technique

1. Inhale and *pull* yourself toward the chair. As you elongate the spine, open the chest and apply a blade squeeze, as in figure 2.
2. Exhale and *push* sideways, as in figure 3. While keeping a blade squeeze, tuck the tailbone and contract the abdominals and ribs to align your spine directly with those well-rooted ischial bones.
3. Inhale into the back of the ribs in this elongated, aligned position.
4. Exhale and *push* with the right hand, as you increase a stronger right-sided blade squeeze. The hips, ribs, chest, shoulders, and head rotate toward the right, as in figure 3.
5. Hold for the count of five as you work to strengthen the muscle around the spinal column. Partly ease the twist to inhale and pull to elongate more.
6. Repeat Technique steps 1-5 five more times. Come out slowly, relax, and repeat with the other side.
7. Repeat the cycle two more times.

Tips

1. Make sure you do *not* arch the lower back too much and lead with the ribs as you twist, as in figure 4. The pelvic triangle is vertical and the head and shoulder girdle are aligned over the pelvic girdle. You work from the pelvis up through the complete spine. Remember the three building blocks of posture. Refer to Proper Body Alignment, section III, chapter 2.
2. In twists, you don't turn from the neck. The rule is to keep the chin in line with the sternum at all times.

Benefits

This exercise massages the internal organs, realigns the vertebrae, relieves tension, and gives a lateral pull to the pelvic region.

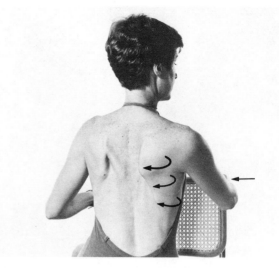

Figure 3

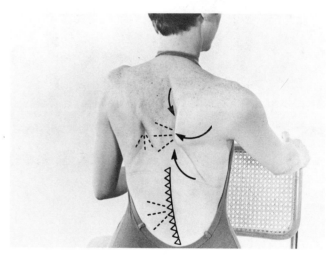

Figure 4
INCORRECT

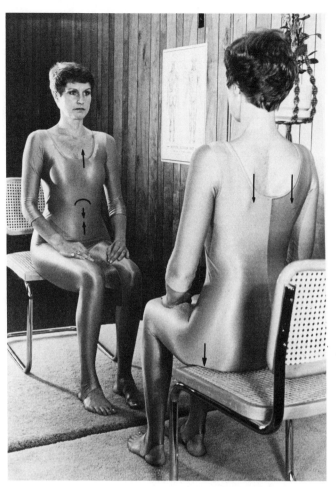

Figure 1

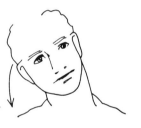

Figure 2

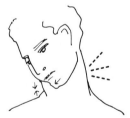

Figure 3
INCORRECT

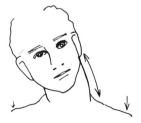

Figure 4

NECK TILT

Props

1. A hard chair placed in front of a mirror.

Body Placement

1. Review Corrective Sitting Habits (section V, chapter 3).
2. Sit with the ischial bones at the edge of the chair. It is very important to maintain a straight, aligned spine throughout this exercise.

Technique

1. While inhaling, elongate the ribs up out of the waist, extend the sternum, and lengthen the neck by shrugging the shoulders back and down. Apply a gentle blade squeeze to align them in place, as in figure 1.
2. While exhaling, tilt your head to the right, and lower your ear toward the shoulder, as in figure 2. Keep the shoulders relaxed and do not raise them.
3. Your eyes should be the same distance from the mirror, *not* as in figure 3, with the head turned.
4. Inhale, sit taller, and maintain the tilt. Exhale as you lower the left shoulder. Feel the muscles tautly pulled, as in figure 4. I want you to feel this strong pull in the neck.
5. Hold the breath out and tilt for the count of five, giving time for the circulation to work.
6. Inhale, ease up on the tilt, and Repeat Technique steps 2-5 five times. Come up and notice that the circulation is improved on the left side of your face and neck.
7. Now, repeat Technique steps 1-6 but tilt to the left. This represents one set. You may do as many as you like—it feels soooo good!

Tips

1. Keep looking straight ahead. The chin doesn't move and the eyes stay vertical.
2. To increase the circulation, it is helpful to frown and squint and then release by moving the scalp and temples.
3. I emphasize the strong stretch in the sternomastoid muscle because it relieves pressure and stimulates the circulation of blood to the brain. One of the causes of headaches is tension buildup, which restricts the blood flow in the head. If headaches or migraines are your problem, do this regularly.
4. Keep in mind the rhythm of your breath as you work within the five tilts per side. Do not rush through the exercise. Take time to feel the benefits and relax inwardly.

Benefits

This exercise is beneficial for migraine headaches and relieves tension and stiffness in the neck.

CHIN CIRCLE

Props

1. A hard chair.

Body Placements

1. Review Corrective Sitting Habits (section V, chapter 3).
2. Sit with the ischial bones at the edge of the chair. Maintain a lifted, elongated spine throughout this exercise.
3. It helps to think you have a pencil in your teeth and are drawing a big, wider-than-possible circle with your pencil (chin). This approach aids in increasing the elongation of the neck and upper back.

Technique

1. Inhale and elongate the neck and sternum with the shoulders down and back. Exhale as you project the chin forward and continue downward to the chest. Tuck in the chin and stretch the back of the neck, as in figure 1. Keep the shoulders down and chest up.
2. While inhaling, extend the sternum and stretch forward from the chin. Continue projecting the chin way up to the ceiling. Exhale and deepen your blade squeeze and lift in the neck, as in figure 2, *not* as in figure 3, with the head dropped back and all hunched up.
3. Inhale and elongate the spine and lift in the back of the neck. Exhale and tilt the spine backward, extending the sternum forward and up, as in figure 4. You are now using the back arching, not the neck, to see overhead. Feel the strength and control in the neck.
4. Inhale, lifting up almost out of your seat. Reach extra high with your chin to make the wide circle and come back to the beginning. Exhale and relax—you made it!
5. Repeat Technique steps 1-4 four more times.

Tips

1. I can't say enough about the importance of good sitting posture. The lower back should not slouch; sit high on the ischial bones.
2. It is *not* important how far you rotate the head. What's important is that you have control of the neck muscles and are strengthening them.

Benefits

This exercise strengthens the neck muscles and relieves tension in the upper thoracic region.

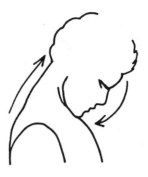

Figure 1

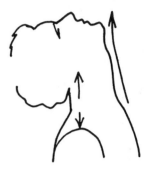

Figure 2

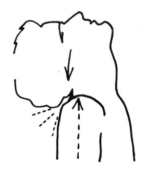

Figure 3
INCORRECT

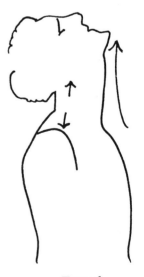

Figure 4

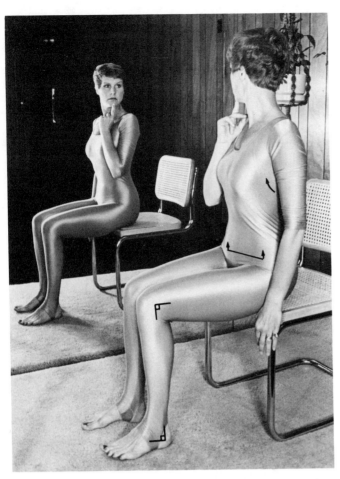

Figure 1

"YES" NECK TURN

Props

1. A firm chair facing sideways in front of a mirror.

Body Placement

1. Review Corrective Sitting Habits (section V, chapter 3).
2. Sit with the ischial bones at the edge of the chair. Maintain a straight aligned spine throughout this exercise.

Technique

1. Inhale, sit tall, and elongate the spine. Stretch your neck as if the chin is resting very lightly on a glass shelf. Place a finger on the chin.
2. Exhale and execute a blade squeeze. With your finger, turn your chin as far as it will go to the right. Face the mirror with your eyes level, as in figure 1, *not* as in figure 2.
3. Inhale as you raise the chin way up. Keep your eyes level and apply a little pressure with your finger to keep the chin rotated as far as it can go, as in figure 3.

4. Exhale as you lower your chin way down. Keep your eyes level and apply pressure with your finger to keep the chin rotated as far as it can go, as in figure 4.
5. Repeat Technique steps 1-4 five more times. Bring the chin back to the center. Turn the chair around and repeat, rotating to the left.

Tips

1. I call this the "Yes" Neck Turn because you are moving up and down, saying a "Yes." Do *not* say a "Maybe" at an angle, as in figure 2.
2. At first, take time to use the mirror, so you can work correctly. After you have learned the movements, you can do without the mirror.

Benefits

This exercise really stimulates and releases tension in the neck muscles and strengthens the alignment in the cervical vertebrae.

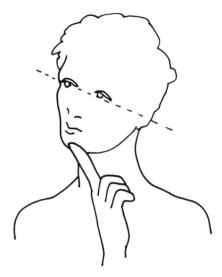

Figure 2
INCORRECT

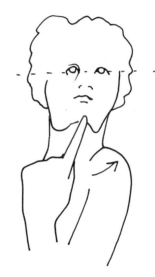

Figure 3

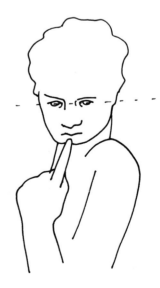

Figure 4

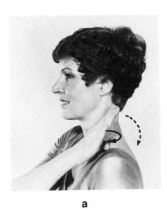
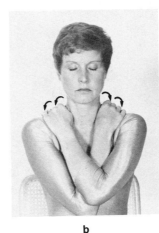

a

b

Figure 1

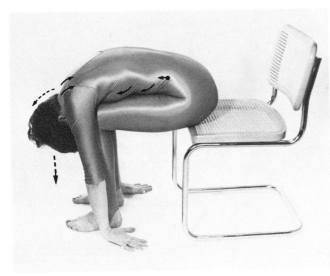

Figure 2

NECK RELAXER

Props

1. A chair.
2. A cervical collar.

Body Placement

1. Review Corrective Sitting Habits (section V, chapter 3).
2. Sit up straight and high on your ischial bones, which are at the edge of your chair.

Technique

1. Inhale, elongate the spine, and extend the sternum.
2. Exhale, rotate the shoulders back and down, apply a blade squeeze, and contract the abdominals.
3. Hold the breath out for five counts.
4. Repeat steps 1-3 five more times.

Variation 1, figure 1, Kneading the Neck

1. Apply Technique steps 1-3, while kneading the neck and shoulder muscles. Tuck the thumb into the palm, and place the thumb knuckle in front of the trapezius muscle and the fingers in back, as in figure 1a. Work the fingers to knead the muscles against the thumb knuckles.
2. The right hand works the left side and the left works the right. You can do both sides at the same time, as in figure 1b.

Variation 2, figure 2, Roll Over Hang

1. Inhale and sit tall. Exhale and slowly lower the head. Tuck under the chin and roll the spine down one vertebra at a time, while rounding the back. Rest the ribs on the thighs.
2. Inhale and elongate the ribs and chest on the thighs. While exhaling, further stretch the top of the head toward the floor and the shoulders up away from the floor, as in figure 2. Really concentrate on stretching the neck and head out of the shoulders. Rotate the head to the left and right, still aiming the *top* of the head toward the floor.
3. Inhale, slowly round your way up, and elongate one vertebra at a time, keeping the arms and head very loose. Feels good, huh—yes, I'm letting you round your back!
4. Repeat Variation 2, steps 1-3 five more times.

Variation 3, figure 3, Hands Clasped Blade Squeeze

1. Apply Technique steps 1-4 with your hands clasped and elbows straight. Work a deeper blade squeeze and extend the sternum, as in figure 3. If you need more room for your arms, sit sideways on the chair.

Variation 4, figure 4, How to Wear a Cervical Collar

1. I see patients who wear a cervical collar lean forward and hang their chin on it, as in figure 4a. This pulls the neck out of alignment and creates a rounded upper back, which adds strain and pinch (pain) in the neck.
2. The collar should not be considered as a crutch but as an aid. The body must maintain proper alignment at all times. Do *not* lean into the collar but elongate the neck up and out of the collar, as in figure 4b. Think that you have a razor sharp edge all along the top of your collar.
3. Apply Technique steps 1-3, while elongating the neck straight up and out of the collar. Now, doesn't that make a big difference? Continue to practice this alignment all the time at work and at home, and you will soon be free of your collar and acquire a stronger, aligned neck.

Tips

1. The single most important relaxer for the neck is to maintain your shoulders down and back away from the ears and draw the head back in like a turtle. Most people extend their neck forward with their shoulders rounded. The ears should line up with the shoulders. Refer to Proper Body Alignment (section III, chapter 2).

Benefits

This exercise relieves and strengthens the neck and shoulder muscles.

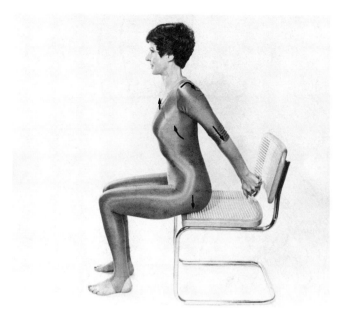

Figure 3

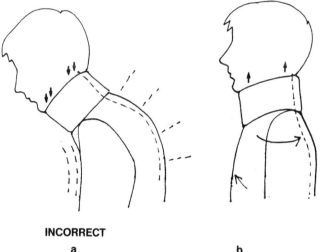

INCORRECT

a   b

Figure 4

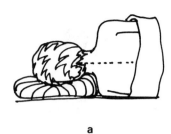

a

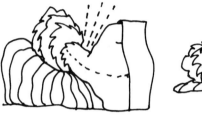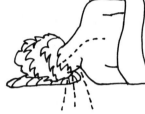

b   c

Figure 1

CORRECTIVE SLEEPING HABITS FOR THE NECK

Props

1. A down or other feathered pillow.

Body Placement

1. Read Corrective Sleeping Habits (section V, chapter 3) to align the rest of the body. Here, we are concentrating only on the head and neck.

Technique for Side Sleeping, figure 1

1. The pillow should be thick and tucked under enough so the neck remains as a straight extension of the spine, as in figure 1a.
2. A pillow that is too high compresses the top side of the neck, as in figure 1b.
3. A pillow that is too low causes compression on the bottom side of the neck, as in figure 1c.

Technique for Stomach Sleeping, figure 2

1. To properly align the neck, the pillow is placed lengthwise with one edge just at the top of the head and the other at the waist, as in figure 2a. With the pillow in this manner, it gives support to the thoracic spine, frees the neck, and there is no more pillow to tuck too much under the head.
2. Do not bunch up the pillow with your arms under it, as in figure 2b. This forces the head and shoulders into the neck, which limits the circulation to the head by compressing the neck.
3. When receiving a massage, and there is no hole in the massage table for your nose, don't turn your head to the side. Fold a towel for under your forehead and roll a bigger towel for under the sternum, as in figure 2c. When your back is massaged, tension can't be jammed into your neck.

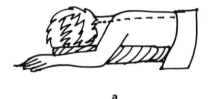

a

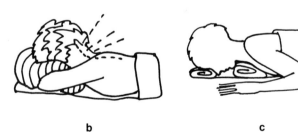

b   c

Figure 2

Technique for Back Sleeping, figures 3 and 4.

1. If you don't use any pillow, the chin is drawn upward, which creates a pinch on the underside of the neck, as in figure 3a. If you sleep this way, and your head and neck are aligned, looking straight up to the ceiling—Good—no need for a pillow. This is rare, though, and in most cases a pillow is needed.

2. In figure 3b, the neck and shoulders are rounded from too high a pillow.

3. Figure 4a shows an aligned neck with a thin pillow under the head and a tightly rolled-up towel, held together with rubber bands, just under the neck. The shoulders are flat on the bed and the head is facing straight up to the ceiling, as in figure 4c.

4. Figure 4b shows my favorite sleeping style. Take the towel, as in figure 4a, and put it inside your pillowcase along one of the long edges. Now, pull the roll to tuck in snugly under the neck, working the head down into the pillow with all the feathers around the head. This insures the alignment. Try this breathing technique: Grab the tips of the pillow with both hands, keeping your elbows on the bed. Inhale and use your elbows to lift up a blade squeeze and the pillow tips in one action. Tuck the roll and pillow comfortably under you. On the exhale, lower your flat shoulder blades down away from your neck. Now, isn't that just heavenly? It might sound complicated; but after a few times, you won't sleep any other way.

Tips

1. The general rule is to keep the shoulders down away from your ears and the neck free (elongated) on all four sides.

2. An old, worn-out pillow works the best. Don't buy a new one, it's too high.

Benefits

The correct Technique insures a relaxed and elongated neck where your circulation can properly flow.

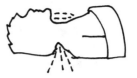

a

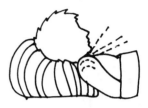

b

Figure 3

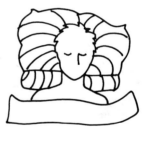

a

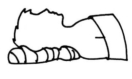

b

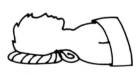

c

Figure 4

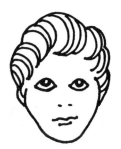

12:00 o'clock

Figure 1

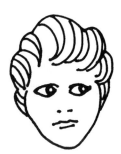

3:00 o'clock

Figure 2

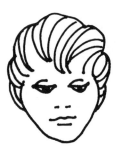

6:00 o'clock

Figure 3

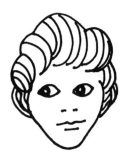

9:00 o'clock

Figure 4

Clock

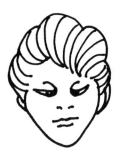

Figure 5

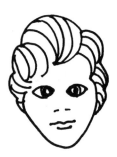

Figure 6

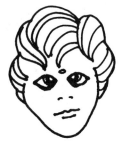

Figure 7
Crossed

EYE EXERCISES

Props

None

Body Placement

1. Sit straight up on the edge of a chair in perfect posture.

Technique, figures 1-4, Clock

1. Look straight ahead and breathe naturally as you do these exercises. Consider your eyes as the hands of a clock.
2. Look way up at 12:00 o'clock (figure 1), left to 3:00 o'clock (figure 2), down to 6:00 o'clock (figure 3), right to 9:00 o'clock (figure 4), and back to 12:00 o'clock (figure 1). Close your eyes, take a deep breath, and rest the eyes after each of the following exercises.
3. Repeat step 2, but go counterclockwise.
4. Repeat the full cycle once more.
5. Proceed to look to the extreme left, as in figure 2. Now switch to the extreme right, as in figure 4. Repeat two more times.
6. Look up as high as you can, as in figure 1, and then down as low as possible, as in figure 3. Repeat two more times.

Technique, figures 5-7, Crossed

1. Continue by looking at the point of your nose, as in figure 5.
2. Cross the eyes, as in figure 6.
3. Finally, look at the spot between your eyebrows (referred to as the third eye and illustrated in figure 7).
4. Close the eyes, take a deep breath, and relax the eyes.
5. Repeat four more times.

Technique, figure 8, Palming

1. Rub the palms of your hands together very fast to create friction and heat. Then, with your eyes closed, place your palms over the eyes, as in figure 8. This relaxes the eyes considerably and can be done after each of these exercises.

Technique, figures 9-12, Not Looking Where You're Going

1. Look way up to the ceiling and keep looking up as you draw the head down, as in figure 9.
2. Close your eyes, take a deep breath, and relax your eyes.
3. Now, look way down at your chest and keep looking down as you draw the head up, as in figure 10.
4. Close your eyes, take a deep breath, and relax your eyes.
5. Proceed to look over your right shoulder and keep looking in that direction as you turn the head to the left, as in figure 11.
6. Close your eyes, take a deep breath, and relax your eyes.
7. End with your eyes looking over your left shoulder and keep looking in that direction as you turn the head to the right, as in figure 12.
8. Close your eyes, take a deep breath, and relax your eyes.
9. Repeat the cycle four more times.

Tips

1. Keep the neck and shoulders relaxed with the head just balancing on top of the aligned spine.
2. After you have mastered all of these exercises, try to do them with your eyes closed.
3. If you feel any eyeball strain, you need to do these exercises. It will soon go away.
4. Remember, to be physically fit, you also must be visually fit.

Benefits

This exercise relieves tension, fatigue, and headaches caused by eyestrain and strengthens the eye muscles.

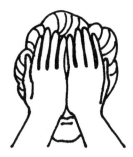

**Figure 8
Palming**

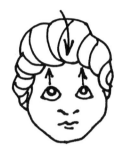

Figure 9

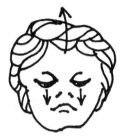

Figure 10

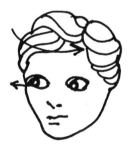

Figure 11

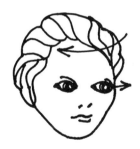

Figure 12

Not Looking Where You're Going

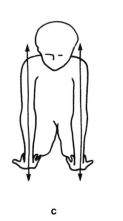

a

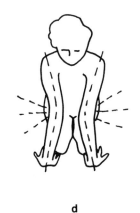

b

c

d

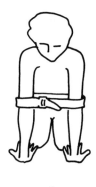

e

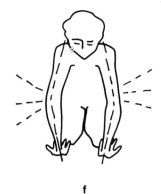

f

Figure 1

7. *Elbows, Wrists, and Hands*

A handshake becomes an ordeal. Turning doorknobs, carrying weights, handling telephones, and closing elevator doors sends arrows of pain searing through your forearm. Brushing your teeth or lifting a cup of tea is an agonizing experience. In tennis, executing a top spin or a backhand and even holding a too-small or too-large racquet handle feels like being struck on the elbow with a hot poker or with the full force of a sledgehammer.

These are all symptoms of an ailment that has become an epidemic in America called "tennis elbow." You certainly needn't be a tennis player to develop tennis elbow. Baseball players, javelin throwers, golfers, football players, and even violinists often suffer identical symptoms. People who use their arms to any great extent in a sport or vocation are susceptible to this disorder. It may produce pain in the lower arm; but the main focus is in the elbow. Tennis elbow results from faulty mechanics. To correct the condition, the weak movement must be found and either adjusted or eliminated. This means the unconditioned elbow should be evaluated and the arm and shoulder alignment reinstated.

When tennis elbow strikes, there are other areas in the arm, shoulder, and upper back about which to be concerned. For example, notice the importance I put on the alignment of the shoulder and neck, in the Tennis Elbow exercise in this chapter. The nerve endings that go down the arm originate in the neck, illustrating the interdependence of the parts of the body. In any movement, think of your body as a total mechanism.

The shoulder blades get a great deal of contraction every time they swing a tennis racket, lift heavy objects, or even close a car door. The trouble is generally accentuated if the movement is consistently one-sided. The shoulder area in the much-used side may be overdeveloped, though the muscles on the other, less-used side are normal or perhaps weaker than normal. This can lead to severe misalignment of the body structure. I often tell people to swing their rackets, clubs, bats, and so forth with the less-used arm to warm-up before the game. But for good insurance, a time should be set aside to properly practice posture throughout playing to develop a better swing. The Tent exercise, explained in section IV, chapter 5, is a good arm strengthener along with the exercises in the chapter.

It is important to understand and execute a properly aligned elbow joint. In exercises such as the Tent, Wrist Stretcher, Chest Opener, and Supine Blade Squeeze, there is weight on or an extension of the whole arm. As a rule, those of you with hyperextended knees have hyperextended elbows as well. Look in a mirror as you execute these exercises. If your elbows bend in the direction of figures 1b, d, or f, you are hyperextending your elbows. Unlock your elbows from the overextended position to what I call an eased elbow as in figures 1a and c. This might feel bent to you but is actually straight. It should release the tension in the joint. Now energy can flow throughout the arm and up into the shoulders and neck. If this feels like an unstable position, use a belt as in figure 1e, which is buckled as wide as the shoulders. The belt is a guide to remind you of what is straight and parallel. As you get stronger in the elbow joint, don't lean into the belt but work away from it so it is slightly loose. The strength in the arm will come from the alignment and the control of your whole shoulder girdle.

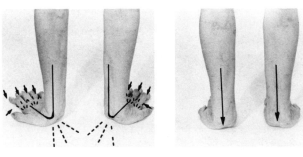

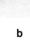

a
INCORRECT

b

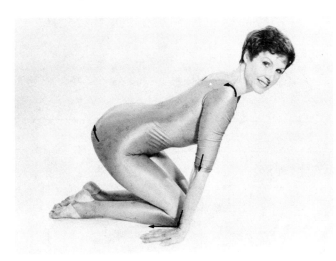

c

Figure 1

Wrist Stretcher

Props
None

Body Placement
1. Kneel on the floor with your knees hip-distance apart.
2. Place your hands beside your knees with the fingers pointing straight back and the knuckles flat, as in figure 1c. Study figures 1a and b.

Technique
1. Inhale, elongate, and lower the sternum to the floor, as you rotate the shoulders back to form a blade squeeze.
2. While exhaling, slowly lower your buttocks to the heels and work a deeper blade squeeze, as in figure 2.
3. Hold the breath out and the position for five counts. Check to see if you look like figure 3, where the shoulders are hunched and not down and/or the elbows are hyperextended. If so, bend the elbows back to make them straight. Now, you will be working your wrists and will *not* weaken your elbows.

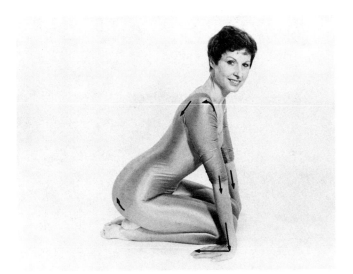

Figure 2

4. Sit back up, as in figure 1c to advance your hands. Slowly work your hands up to where you can sit down with the fingertips at the knee, as in figure 4.
5. Repeat Technique steps 1-3 at each level until you achieve five wrist stretches.

Tips

You do not have to go to the final position to feel you have accomplished the stretch. I'm more interested in the quality of work. Are you sitting back on your heels with your back straight and knuckles flat? Your fingers should be straight back, *not* at an angle.

Benefits

This exercise is excellent stretch for the wrist and arms.

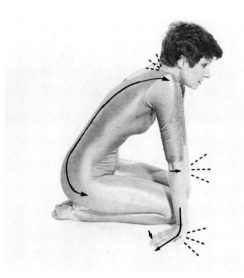

Figure 3
INCORRECT

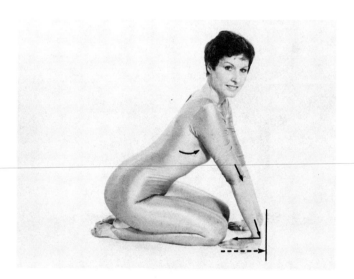

Figure 4

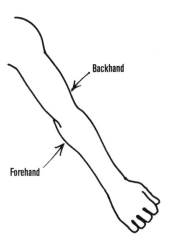

Backhand

Forehand

Figure 1

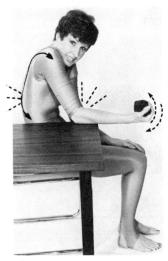

Figure 2

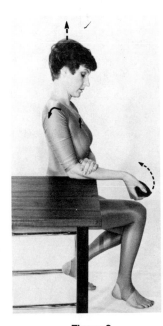

Figure 3

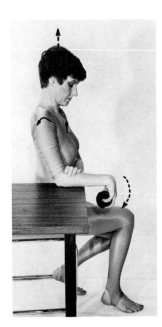

Figure 4

TENNIS ELBOW EXERCISE

Props

1. A chair by a table..
2. A three- or five-pound weight.

Body Placement

1. Sit straight up with the ischial bones on the edge of the chair and maintain a blade squeeze as you lift the weight.
2. Study figure 1 to evaluate your pain and problem.
3. If you are in pain, first practice this exercise with *no* weight. Take caution to align the body and shoulders. After some of the pain has dissipated, you can add some weight.

Technique

1. While inhaling, extend your sternum and sit tall with your ribs next to your elbow. Lay your arm flat on the table and let your hand extend over the edge.
2. Exhale, contract your abdominals, and apply a blade squeeze. Keep the shoulder in line with the elbow, *not* out of line, as in figure 2.

Variation 1

1. For the front wrist curls, your palm is facing up, as in figure 3.
2. Use Technique steps 1 and 2 to execute the correct alignment. Inhale when your hand is in the extreme up or down position (at rest). Exhale during the work phases of the lifts.
3. Lift your hand up and down ten times, trying to move your wrist through the greatest range of motion.
4. Repeat three times.

Variation 2

1. For the back wrist curls, your palms are facing down, as in figure 4.
2. Repeat Variation 1, steps 2 and 3.

Tips

1. The symptoms of tennis elbow may be caused from overuse, incorrect playing habits, or racquet size, to name a few. Learn good mechanics and a smooth, relaxed stroke.
2. Use your best judgment on how many repeats you do and how much weight you use. Remember, tennis elbow is an *overuse* injury, which needs rest and tender loving care.

Benefits

This exercise is an excellent exercise for tennis elbow.

SPIDER HAND PRESS

Props

1. A table or flat surface.

Body Placement

1. Proper body alignment should be maintained when sitting or standing.

Technique

1. Inhale and press both palms and fingers together, as in figure 1a. While exhaling, draw the tips of the fingers down by bending outward only the middle knuckles, as in figure 1b. Keep the other two joints pressing into each other. Repeat this motion up and down five times and rest.
2. Repeat Technique step 1 but with the palms apart and pressing only the fingers and big knuckles, as in figures 2a and b.
3. Stand up beside a table. Inhale and apply a blade squeeze, while pressing the whole hand flat on a table with the wrist at a right angle, as in figure 3a.
4. While exhaling, keep your hand pressing down as you slide the tips of the fingers in bringing up the middle knuckle, as in figure 3b. Repeat five more times. If you are having difficulty with this exercise, repeat it but use your hands as suggested in figures 4a and b. For some of you, it may hurt, but keep doing it—it's the best thing for these joints.

Tips

This is an exercise you can do at any time. I encourage you to do it many times a day if you have cold or tight joints.

Benefits

This exercise is excellent for arthritic fingers and hands. It also stimulates cold hands.

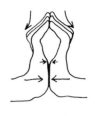
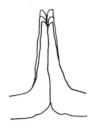

a   b

Figure 1

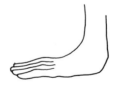
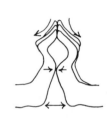

a   b

Figure 2

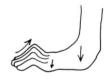
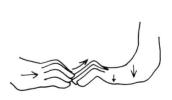

a   b

Figure 3

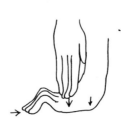

a   b

Figure 4

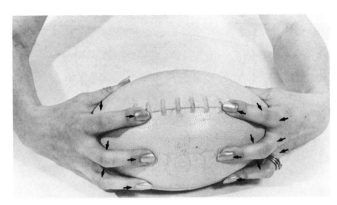

Figure 1

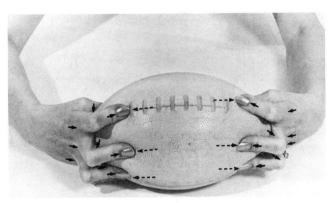

Figure 2

a   b

Figure 3

FINGER EXERCISES

Props

1. A Nerf football.

Body Placement

1. Sit straight up on the edge of a chair in perfect posture.
2. As you practice these finger exercises, it is important that you maintain an erect upper body. Do not slouch. The blade squeeze and proper shoulder placement assists in the energy and strength you can apply to your hands.

Technique

1. Inhale and wrap your fingers around the ends of the football. Bring the football deep into your hand so your fingers are outstretched around it, as in figure 1.
2. Exhale and apply a blade squeeze, while contracting your abdominals. Squeeze down into the football to bend down and inward the first finger joints nearest the nails.
3. Hold the breath out and the press for a count of five.
4. Inhale and elongate your correct posture. While exhaling, slowly start to draw the bent, squeezing fingers to the ends of the football, as in figure 2. The closer you squeeze to the smaller ends of the football, the deeper the bend in the finger joints. Hold for five counts.
5. Repeat Technique steps 1-4 five more times and do this exercise often daily.

Technique for Opening and Closing Fist, figure 3

1. Inhale, sit tall, and outstretch your fingers in both hands wide open, as in figure 3a.
2. While exhaling, contract the abdominals and squeeze the blades. Slowly, isometrically draw your fingers in, bending one joint at a time into a tight fist, as in figure 3b. Repeat ten more times.

Technique for Pulling Fingers, figure 4

1. Inhale, sit tall, and grasp your left thumb with your right hand, as in figure 4. Pull the thumb to free the joint.
2. While exhaling, contract the abdominals and squeeze the blades. Gently twist the left thumb toward the body and then away from the body. Pull the thumb again, hold, and release.
3. Repeat Technique steps 1 and 2. Proceed with this same method with all ten fingers.

Figure 4

Technique for Bending the Wrist, figure 5

1. Inhale, sit tall, and draw your fingers straight up, as in figure 5a. It is helpful to press the hands against a wall, making a right angle at the wrist. Hold for five counts.
2. Exhale, contract the abdominals, and squeeze the blades. Draw your fingers down to make a right angle, as in figure 5b. Hold for five counts.
3. Repeat Technique steps 1 and 2 ten times.

a   b

Figure 5

Technique for Praying Hand Press, figure 6

1. Inhale, sit tall, and press the heels, palms, and all the knuckles together, as in figure 6a.
2. Exhale, contract the abdominals and squeeze the blades. Pull apart, as far as they will go, only the heels of the hands and palms, as in figure 6b. Keep all three knuckles of each finger pressing against each other.
3. Hold w-i-d-e apart for three long breaths.

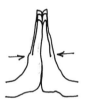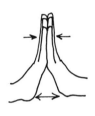

a   b

Figure 6

Technique for Individual Finger, figure 7

1. Inhale, sit tall, and stretch the fingers out wide.
2. Exhale, contract the abdominals, and squeeze the blades. Slowly roll each finger down separately toward the palm of the hand, as in figure 7. Concentrate on not moving the upright fingers at all.
3. Repeat Technique steps 1 and 2 for each finger of both hands. If this is difficult for you, repeat four more times.

Tips

1. While you are doing these exercises, concentrate on keeping the rest of the body aligned and relaxed.
2. Do not let tension creep up the arm and into the neck. If this should happen, start all over by relaxing the arm and neck.

Benefits

This exercise helps arthritic fingers and hands. It also stimulates cold hands.

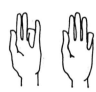

Figure 7

Section V

Bodysense Total Fitness Program

1. *Daily Dozen Routine*
   Levels I and II
2. *Relaxation Technique*
3. *Daily Living Habits*
4. *Bodysense and Beyond*

1. Daily Dozen Routine
Levels I and II

The Daily Dozen Routine should not be used without reading this book from the beginning to understand the Bodysense Method. I want you to examine yourself and be able to know your body's pattern, it's weaknesses and strengths. To use the Bodysense Method, you have to know your own unique posture, be able to draw it into proper alignment, and execute the exercises with balance and rhythmic breathing.

The Daily Dozen Routine has been put together for your convenience; but if you find yourself rushed, please do only what you can in the correct manner. Take time for some deep breaths and relaxation and save the remaining portion for the next day. As you become more relaxed and flexible, you will be able to do more exercises.

Don't just practice the exercises you do well. At least two times a week, add the particular exercise on which your body needs to work. Remember to work at your own level, edge, rhythm, and balance. You then can keep yourself aligned and fit into the future.

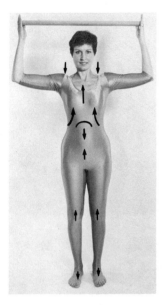

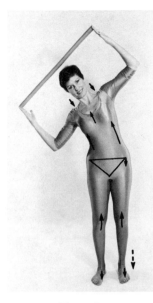

Figure 1 **Figure 2**

**Level I
Blade Squeeze**

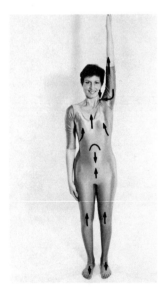

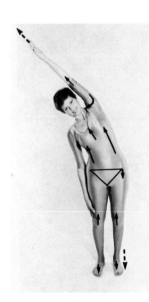

Figure 3 **Figure 4**

**Level II
Lateral Stretch**

SIDE STRETCH

Props
Level I. A 2½-foot long pole.
Level II. None.

Body Placement, Levels I and II
1. Stand with your feet parallel, hip-distance apart, with the kneecaps raised and feet well-rooted to the floor.
2. Keep the pubic bone forward in line with the hipbones to form the pelvic triangle.
3. Shoulders should remain down away from the ears with a squaring off of the shoulders into a blade squeeze.

Level I. Clasp the pole with your palms facing forward. Keep the pole centered with your head and elbows bent at shoulder level.

Level II. Raise one arm up beside your ear. To free the shoulder joint, bend the elbow to start off, then work the stretch from the ribs as you straighten the arm.

Technique
1. While inhaling, ground the feet and stengthen the legs straight as you elongate the spine.
2. While exhaling, vertically tuck the pelvic triangle and contract the abdominals. Keep your shoulders down. Tilt to the right, reaching only upward. Do not fold at the waist.
3. Hold for five counts.
4. Still tilted, inhale and press the left foot deeper, while elongating the whole side of the body.
5. While exhaling, stabilize the pelvic triangle and continue to tilt upward and diagonally.
6. Hold for five counts. Repeat one more cycle. Come out of the tilt and repeat with the left side. Repeat four times with each side.

Tips
1. Keep your shoulders squared off away from your ears.
2. Maintain an aligned shoulder girdle, while stretching from the hips to elbows. The tilt does *not* come from the neck.
3. As you tilt, the legs and feet continue to reach downward to ground yourself.

Reference
Level I. Blade Squeeze with Pole, section IV, chapter 6.
Level II. Lateral Stretch, section IV, chapter 5.

STANDING FORWARD BEND

Props
Level I. A 2½-foot long pole.
Level II. None.

Body Placement
Stand with your toes raised and place your feet from hip-distance to three feet apart. Keep your knees bent and feet rooted to the floor

Level I. Place the pole on your back at the waist and your hands around the buttocks with your fingers on the ischial bones, as in figure 1.

Level II. Place your hands around the buttocks with your fingers on the ischial bones, as in figure 3.

Technique
1. While inhaling, elongate the spine and extend the sternum. Roll your shoulders back and away from your ears.
2. Exhale and lift up the skin under your fingers, as you work to straighten your legs. Keep the weight of your body more into the balls of the feet so you won't hyperextend your knees.
3. Hold the breath out and stretch for five counts.
4. Repeat steps 1-3 five times.

Tips
Level I

1. Keep your spine and elbows away from the pole. *Don't* hang on the pole.
2. You do *not* have to force your leg straight. When bent, if you feel the stretch—hold that level.
3. Once you can maintain rotation in the hips, hold onto your ribs to keep the elongation in the spine, as in figure 2.

Level II

1. When bending your knees, bring your ribs down onto the thighs and keep them together, as you work at straightening the legs.
2. Do *not* straighten your leg if your ribs come off the thighs.
3. When your legs are straight bring your hand up from under to further lift the ischial bones, as in figure 4.

Reference
Level I. Standing Forward Bend with Pole, section IV, chapter 5.
Level II. Forward Bending Hamstring Stretch, section IV, chapter 5.

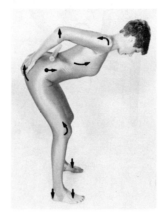
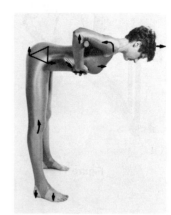

Figure 1   **Figure 2**
Level I
Standing Forward Bend with Pole

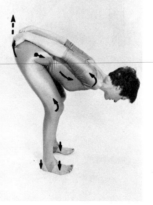
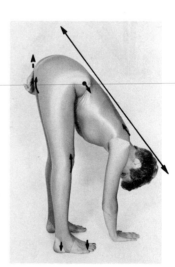
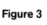

Figure 3

Figure 4
Level II
Forward Bending Hamstring Stretch

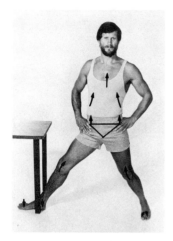

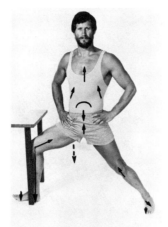

Figure 1 **Figure 2**

Level I

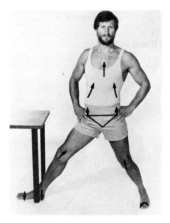

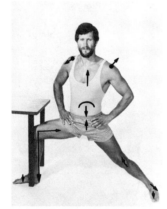

Figure 3 **Figure 4**

Level II

FRONT FACING PLUNGE

Props

1. An outside corner or furniture.

Body Placement

1. Stand with your feet three to four feet apart with the right ankle at the edge, as in figures 1 and 3.
2. With your hands on your hips, pivot, and turn the right foot out and the left foot in.
3. Both knees should line up with the feet and the kneecaps should be raised. Adjust your hips, while working your pelvic triangle to be vertical.

Technique

1. Inhale with your feet firmly rooted. Raise your kneecaps and elongate your spine, while keeping the shoulders down.
2. While exhaling, contract the abdominals and tuck the tailbone to bring the pelvic triangle vertical, as in figures 1 and 3.
3. Inhale and sustain the lift. Exhale with firmness in the legs and bend the right knee to the corner, as in figures 2 and 4. Hold the breath and position for five counts.
4. Repeat steps 1-3 continually as you work toward a right angle with the right leg. After five breaths, come out and repeat with the left leg.

Tips

Level I. Go as far as you can *only* if you can maintain the pelvic triangle and a vertical spine. Do *not* force lowering for the sake of your balance and control.

Level II. As you are able to lower toward a right angle, you may have to slide your left foot further back. Keep your feet firmly rooted.

Reference

Front Facing Plunge, section IV, chapter 2.

SIDE FACING PLUNGE

Props

1. A leg of a table or an outside corner.

Body Placement

1. Stand with your feet three to four feet apart. Pivot the hips and legs, turning to face and line up with the right foot against the edge, as in figure 1.
2. There should be an imaginary hip-width space between the inside edges of both feet.
3. Place your hands on your hips to steer and monitor a vertical pelvic triangle. While bending the left knee, rotate your left hip forward to line up even with the right hip, as in figure 1. If the hips don't line up, bring your left foot in closer.

Technique

1. While inhaling, press the right foot down and lift the toes, arch, and kneecap. Elongate your spine up out of the waist.
2. Exhale and bend your right knee to line up with the corner. Bend your left knee to draw the left hip even with the right hip, as in figure 1.
3. Inhale and elongate. While exhaling, rotate the tailbone to draw the pubic bone forward, which makes the pelvic triangle completely vertical.
4. Exhale and contract your abdominals. Keep the pelvic triangle level and the left and right hips in line with each other, as you work to straighten out the left leg, as in figure 2. Try to lower your heel to the floor without moving your left hip.
5. Repeat Technique steps 3 and 4 six times. Work into an aligned, balanced position.
6. Come out and repeat with the left leg.

Tips

Level I. If it is difficult to level off your hips, draw the left foot in closer and balance up on the ball of the foot. Do not let your left hip drop back when working the left heel toward the floor.

Level II. If you have accomplished Level I with your body aligned and the left heel on the floor, start over with Technique step 1 by placing your feet 3½ or 4 feet apart, as in figure 3, and continue with Technique steps 1-5. Don't let your right knee go beyond the post, as in figure 3. Keep the knee over the ankle, as in figure 4.

Reference

Side Facing Plunge, section IV, chapter 5.

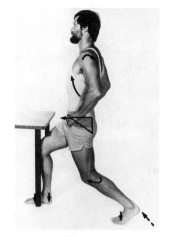 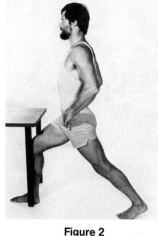

Figure 1	Figure 2

Level I

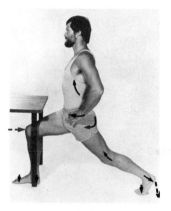 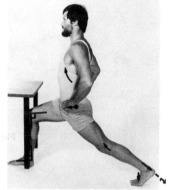

Figure 3	Figure 4

Level II

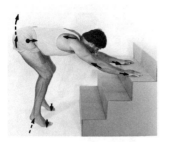

Figure 1

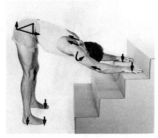

Figure 2

Level I

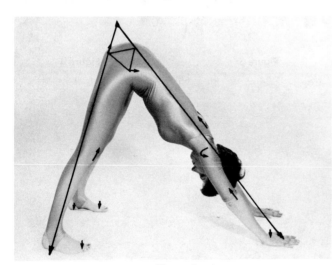

Figure 3

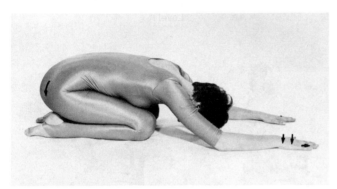

Figure 4
Level II

THE TENT

Props

Level I. A stairway.
Level II. The floor.

Body Placement

Level I. Kneel in front of the stairs with your knees hip-width apart and extend the arms shoulder-width apart. Stretch back away from the stairs, so your hands are on the edge of the appropriate step, while keeping your buttocks over, your heels, as in figure 2.

Level II. Kneel, sit back on your heels, bend forward, and outstretch your arms and hands, as in figure 3.

Technique

1. Inhale and lift your buttocks toward the ceiling. Balance up on the balls of your feet. While exhaling, completely straighten your arms and apply a push on the step or floor to feel strength in the arms.
2. While inhaling, elongate the spine and lower your chest toward the floor. Squeeze your shoulder blades together and work a straight back, as in figure 1.
3. While exhaling, push away and draw your ears in line with your arms. The buttocks continues to rotate upward.
4. Inhale and keep your knees bent in both Levels I and II. Elongate the arms and spine in both directions, lengthening from the hands to the tailbone.
5. Exhale and keep your ischial bones rotated upward. Straighten your legs by raising your kneecaps, while being up high on the balls of your feet.
6. Inhale and continue to rotate your ischial bones. Do *not* move your arms or spine. Exhale and lower your heels as you attempt to raise your toes to keep the arches lifted, as in figures 2 and 4.
7. Hold the breath out as you work deeper into the position.
8. Repeat Technique steps 4-7 five times.

Tips

Level I. If you can keep your arms, spine, and legs straight, as in figure 2, reach for a lower step but adjust your Body Placement accordingly.

Level II. Make sure you don't sink heaviness in the arms. Push down into the floor but elongate the arm, spine, and legs upward, and backward, as if someone was pulling you up.

Reference

The Tent, section IV, chapter 5.

STANDING BENT LEG TWIST

Props

1. A chair.
2. A wall.

Body Placement

1. Stand with your heels three inches away from the wall and hip-distance apart.
2. Place the right hand on top of the backrest of the chair and bend your elbow. The left arm is bent back so the hand can feel for the smooth groove of the recessed spine, as in figure 1.
3. Bend your right knee and press (screw) the two ischial bones to the wall.
4. The hand placement on the chair depends on your flexibility. Keep feeling your back for a smooth groove. Study the hand and spine positions of figures 1-4.

Technique

1. Inhale and elongate the spine with the two ischial bones (screwed) to the wall as the base of the twist.
2. Exhale and rotate the right shoulder back and down. Pull the elbow behind you and apply a deeper blade squeeze.
3. Inhale and continue to elongate in *both* directions from your head to your ischial bones, as well as having your feet firmly grounded into floor.
4. Exhale and, from the downward action in the legs, rotate the ischial bones up the wall. Start the twist from the base of the hips and screwed ischial bones into a smooth, straight groove—feel for it with your hands. Keeping your chest in line with the sternum makes the neck act as a continuation of the twist.
5. Partly ease out of the twist to elongate more. Repeat Technique steps 1-5 four times. Come out of the twist and repeat with the other side.

Tips

Level I

1. You *must* maintain the elongation before each rotation to employ the proper distance in the discs. This insures a healthy rotation of the vertebrae.
2. I know the bent-leg ischial bone wants to come off the wall but don't let it.

Level II. In executing a twist properly, don't just turn and twist from your weakest or most flexible areas. The legs and spine must be grounded and stabilized by working the two ischial bones (screwed) into the wall.

Reference

Standing Bent Leg Twist, section IV, chapter 5.

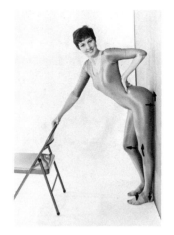

Figure 1   **Figure 2**

Level I

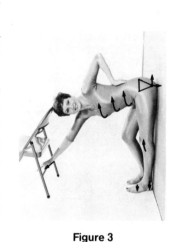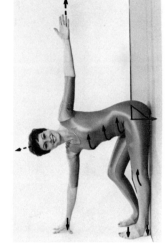

Figure 3   **Figure 4**

Level II

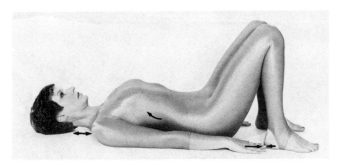

Figure 1

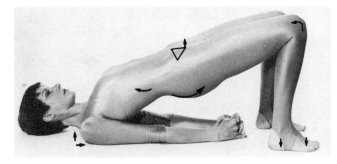

Figure 2
Level I

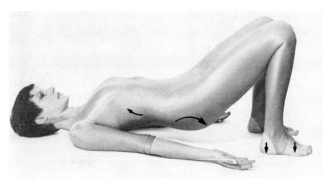

Figure 3

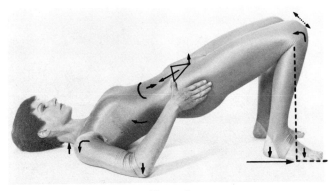

Figure 4
Level II

BURNING BUTT

Props

None

Body Placement

1. Lie down and bend your knees so your feet are parallel and hip-distance apart. Your heels should come to the tips of your fingers.
2. Adjust your head so your neck is elongated, as in figure 1.

Technique

1. Inhale and press your feet into the floor—all eight tires (balls and heels) worth. Exhale and roll the buttocks up, leading with the rotated action of the tailbone.
2. Inhale and, with your arms straight on the floor, clasp your hands beneath you and squeeze your shoulder blades together, while walking your shoulders in together and away from your neck. Your cervical spine should be free and lifted completely off the floor, as in figure 2.
3. Keeping your chest up, exhale and lower your hips as if to sit down, as in figure 3.
4. Inhale and extend the sternum. While exhaling, contract the abdomen and rib cage where the frontal hipbones and floating ribs draw toward each other. Put your hands on your hips, as in figure 4.
5. Inhale into the back of the ribs. While exhaling, contract the abdomen and rotate the tailbone in an attempt to kick the pubic bone higher than your hipbones. Your fingers are pulling your hips toward your waist and down, as in figure 4.
6. Repeat step 5 three more times to increase your rotation.
7. Come down and rest.
8. Repeat the exercise three more times, taking seven breaths to execute the Burning Butt.

Tips
Level I

1. Make sure your cervical spine is off the floor; so squeeze those arms and blades together.
2. Keep your knees vertically in line with your ankles and keep pressing the feet (eight tires) into the floor.

Level II

1. Do not arch your back. You should have an inclined spine. Feel for the smooth groove with your fingers.
2. If you tend to open your knees wider than your ankles, put a belt around your thighs to keep the correct distance.

3. The tendency is to come forward with the knees, bringing them out of their right angle, as in figure 4. Keep yourself in a right angle with the dotted line.

Reference

Burning Butt, section IV chapter 2.

KNEELING THIGH TILT

Props

Level I. A chair.
Level II. None.

Body Placement

1. Kneel with your knees and feet hip-distance apart.
2. Keep the knees hip-distance apart, but squeeze them together in their skin to bring them up on top of the kneecaps, as in figure 1.

Level I. Place the palms of your hands down on the chair, as in figure 2. Keep your arms straight and your chest lifted.

Level II. Place your hands on the front of the thighs, tuck in your chin, and shrug your shoulders forward, as in figure 3.

Technique

1. Inhale and elongate the sternum. While exhaling, contract your abdomen and rotate your hips by tucking your tailbone to push the pubic bone forward.
2. Inhale and keep your pubic bone forward and the sternum elongated. Exhale slowly and tilt your body, as in figures 2 and 4. Hold for a count of six. Come up on the inhale.
3. As you are in the tilt and holding the position, you are continually tightening up the rotation of the pubic bone forward, as well as squeezing the knees.
4. Repeat steps 1-3 five more times.

Tips

1. The clue in this tilt is to keep the knees squeezing together, which tightens the buttocks and the continual rotation in the hips.
2. Don't let your head arch back; keep the chin tucked in.
3. If you feel discomfort in the shoulders, the chair may be too high for you. Use something lower, but don't arch your back. Keep the spine and arms straight.

Reference

Kneeling Thigh Tilt, section IV, chapter 2.

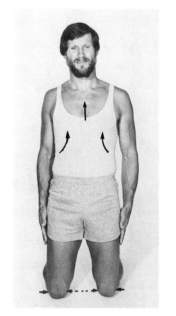

Figure 1

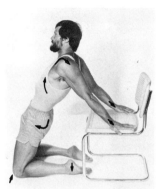

Figure 2

Level I

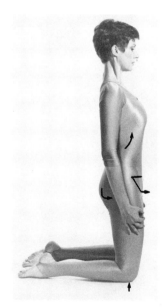

Figure 1   **Figure 2**

Level II

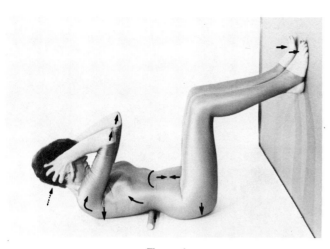

Figure 1

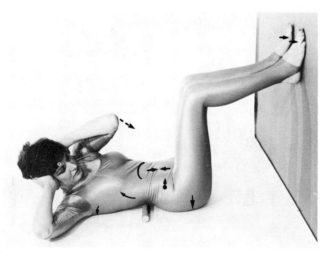

Figure 2
Level I

SACRUM BALANCE WITH ROLL-UP

Props

1. A one-inch thick by twelve-inch long pole

Body Placement

1. Lie down. Place your feet on the wall so your leg forms a right angle.
2. The feet stay flat on the wall.
3. Place your hands to cup your ears, with your elbows toward the knees, as in figure 1.

Technique

1. While inhaling, elongate your ribs up and out of the waist. Anchor on the sacrum with the pole comfortably under your back.
2. While exhaling, contract your abdomen and draw only the head and tops of your shoulders, not the blades, off the floor, as in figure 1.
3. Hold the breath out for six counts, while dipping the tailbone toward the floor. Push slightly with your feet to further contract the abdomen, while keeping your ribs up and out of the waist. Still keeping off of the pole, balance on your sacrum and maintain a level pelvic triangle.
4. Lower your head and shoulders. Repeat until you can accomplish keeping the pelvic triangle level and abdomen from popping.

Level I

1. Repeat Technique steps 1-3. Upon holding the breath out maintain your anchored abdominals and cross your left elbow over the right side, as in figure 2.
2. Dipping the tailbone down keeps the pelvic triangle level, even while twisting the upper body.
3. Rest your head. Repeat with the opposite elbow.
4. Repeat five more times.

Level II, figure 3

1. Repeat Level 1, steps 1 and 2.
2. While reaching over with your left elbow and feeling secure in the abdominal balance, lift your right foot *only* one inch off the wall, as in figure 3.
3. Hold the balance for a count of six and still remain off the pole.
4. Rest your head and foot. Repeat with the opposite side.
5. Repeat three more times.

Level II, figure 4

1. Repeat Level 2, steps 1-3.
2. With properly secured balance, lift your second foot *only* one inch off the wall. Now, you have two feet off the wall, as in figure 4.
3. Rest your head and feet. Repeat with the opposite side.
4. Repeat three more times.

Tips

1. This is a graduated exercise. So remember, it's the quality of the doing that counts.
2. As the exercise becomes effortless, you may add ankle weights and do more repetitions.
3. At all times the pole should remain comfortable and the abdominals must not pop but be firm and flat.

Reference

Sacrum Balance with Roll-Up, section IV, chapter 4.

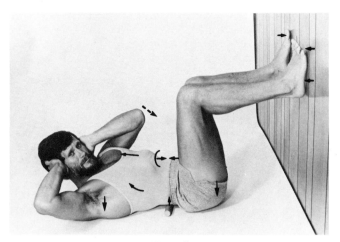

Figure 3

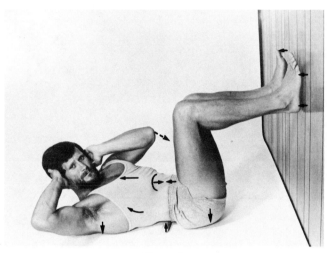

Figure 4
Level II

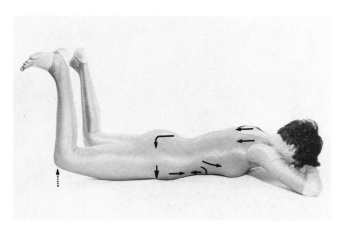

Figure 1

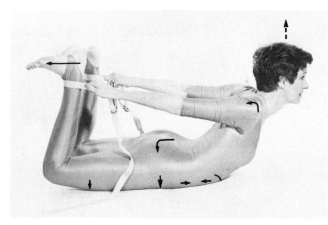

Figure 2
Level I

THE BOW

Props

1. Optional, two belts.

Body Placement

1. Lie on your stomach with your hands under your forehead. Shrug your shoulders down away from your ears.
2. Knees are hip-distance apart and your legs remain parallel with the feet flexed so the soles face the ceiling.
3. Rotate your tailbone down and under. Contract the abdominals, so the navel lifts inward. The pubic bone and frontal hipbones are the foundation of this exercise.

Technique

1. Inhale and elongate the spine and ribs up out of the waist.
2. While exhaling, rotate the tailbone down and under and contract the abdominals to anchor the pelvic-triangle foundation.
3. Inhale and elongate without drawing the shoulders up; they should remain rotated in a blade squeeze. While exhaling, stabilize your foundation and raise the thighs off the floor, as in figure 1. They will not come up too high, but notice the stength and control in the lower back.
4. Hold for a count of five. Repeat one more breath to reinforce the stabilization of your foundation. Come down and rest.

Level I, figure 2

1. If you find it difficult to grab your ankles, looping two belts at the ankles will give you the length you need. Hold onto the belts, with the shoulders shrugged back and down away from the ears into a tight shoulder blade squeeze, as in figure 2.
2. Inhale and elongate the spine forward and upward. While exhaling, stabilize your foundation by contracting the abdominals and ribs. Keep the thighs on the floor to create a bowstring effect with your arms taut.
3. Inhale and increase the elongation. While exhaling, press the ankles into the belt and stabilize your foundation and balance by working the ribs off the floor.
4. Hold for five counts. Use this breathing pattern for two more rounds. Continuously lift the spine higher. Come down and rest.

Level II, figure 3

1. Repeat Level I, steps 2-4, but grab your ankles with your hands, as in figure 3.
2. Don't push your abdominals into the floor; contract them inward. The neck extends up out of the shoulders but is also relaxed. Keep the bowstring effect between the shoulders and feet.

Level II, figure 4

1. To raise both ends at the same time, hold onto your ankles, inhale, and elongate the spine forward and upward.
2. While exhaling, rotate the tailbone to stabilize your pelvic foundation by contracting the abdominals and ribs. Keep your pubic bone rooted to the floor.
3. Inhale and increase the elongation and tautness in the arms and shoulders.
4. Exhale and, with a stabilized foundation, reach to the ceiling with the top of the head and soles of the feet, as in figure 4.
5. Hold for five counts. Use this breathing pattern for two more rounds. Continuously reach higher. Come down and relax.

Tips

1. There should be no need to round your back for relief if the exercise is done correctly. This is a good way to monitor the quality of your work. Each of my exercises is complete in itself. You should not need relief, if you do them properly.
2. Do *not* swing yourself up with momentum—that is *not* working from control.
3. Keep your legs parallel. I know they want to swing out, but work more from the hips and tighten the pelvic foundation.

Reference

The Bow, section IV, chapter 5.

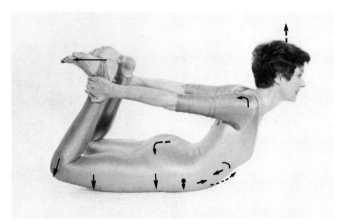

Figure 3

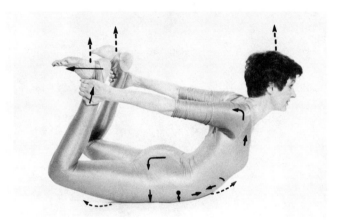

Figure 4
Level II

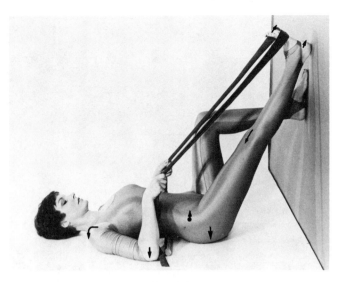

Figure 1

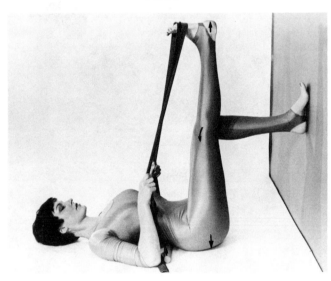

Figure 2

HAMSTRING STRETCH AT WALL

Props

1. A wall.
2. Two long neckties tied together at the wide end and measuring approximately eight feet long.
3. A one-inch thick by twelve-inch long pole under the waist.

Body Placement

1. Lie down, with both your feet on the wall and your knees bent to form a right angle, as is the left leg in figure 1.
2. Place the wide part of the tie against the ball of your foot. With your elbows on the floor, slide your right heel up the wall. Keep your toes toward your face.

Technique

1. Inhale and elongate the spine off the pole. With your toes toward your face, grip the tie taut and push the ball of the foot into the tie.
2. Exhale and tighten your leg straight by lifting the kneecap toward the thigh (not locked back).
3. Hold your position and repeat a complete breath. Make sure your spine is not pressing into the pole and you are anchored on the tailbone edge of the sacrum.
4. On the third exhale, contract your abdomen and balance on the sacrum, while advancing forward. Hold for five counts.

Level I

1. Inhale and elongate the spine off the pole, while anchoring on the sacrum.
2. Exhale, contract your abdomen, and tighten your leg straight.
3. Inhale again. Without pulling your leg with the tie, exhale and use the abdominals to advance your legs forward in stages.
4. Hold your leg there with the tie. Use it as leverage to inhale and elongate off the pole.
5. Hold the leg at each stage for a count of five.
6. Make sure you dip the tailbone downward and keep the sacrum firm on the floor.
7. Repeat steps 1-6, until your leg is *free* to balance, as in figure 2.

8. Return your leg to the right-angle position.
9. Repeat with your other leg.

Level II

1. Slide out so your right heel is where the floor and wall meet, as in figure 3.
2. Take the pole away but keep space under your waist to maintain a level pelvic triangle, even as the leg advances.
3. Place the tie across the back of your left foot. Hold the tie with both hands where your arms can be straight and shoulder blades toward each other flat on the floor, as in figure 3.
4. Repeat steps 1-6 in Level I without the pole, but work to keep a smaller space under your waist.
5. Work at your own level. Don't push to be as figure 4. Take three long breaths into each advancement of the leg, giving time to warm the muscles.
6. Keep working the ball and heel of your right foot into the wall. It helps to keep the pelvic triangle level.
7. Hold the final position for five counts.
8. Return your leg to the floor.
9. Repeat with your other leg.

Tips

1. Do *not* go on to Level II unless your legs can be extended completely straight.
2. If your legs cannot straighten, continue to take about five breaths to work it—but don't force. Breathe into it.
3. If your legs are tight, there is a tendency to roll up your buttocks and press the spine into the pole. *Do not do that.*
4. Keep your spine off the pole and your tailbone end of the sacrum anchored to the floor. Work from where your leg is straight. Your hamstring will become more flexible.
5. As you advance your raised leg forward, make sure you don't roll your thighs out to the side. Keep your hips even and level—a horizontal pelvic triangle. It helps to keep working the sit bones toward each other.

Reference

Hamstring Strech at Wall, section IV, chapter 2.

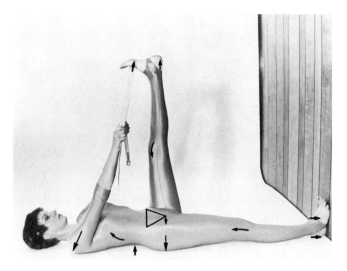

Figure 3

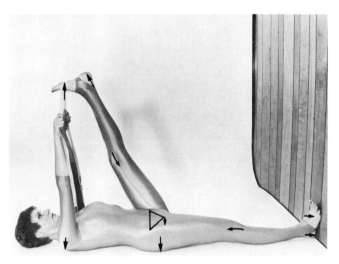

Figure 4

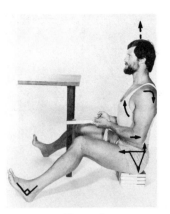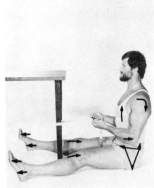

| **Figure 1** | **Figure 2** |

Level I
Sitting Up on the Ischial Bones

SITTING EXERCISES

Props

1. A table.
2. **Level I**, one belt.
   Level II, two belts.
3. Books or blankets.

Body Placement

1. Review the exercise Sitting Up on the Ischial Bones (section IV, chapter 3) to understand the best position for the alignment of your pelvic girdle and spine.
2. Sit close to the table so the post (leg) is between your legs, as in figure 1. Wrap a belt around the post and hold both straps in your left hand. This frees the right hand to feel the back to check if you are working correctly.

Technique

1. Inhale, elongate, and extend the front of the body, while grounding on your ischial bones.
2. Exhale and secure your alignment (smooth groove) and firm foundation (grounded).
3. Hold the breath out for a count of six, as you continue to rotate the frontal hipbones forward and advance with the spine.
4. Repeat steps 1-3 five more times. Rest.

Level I

1. Repeat Technique steps 1-4, using the leverage of pulling the belts for elongation and extension. Make sure your elbows work behind your ribs, as in figure 1.
2. Once the spine is balanced straight up upon your ischial bones, work at straightening your legs without letting the spine pop out.
3. When you accomplish getting the spine and legs straight, start removing one book at a time, until you can sit as in figure 2.
4. Do not sacrifice your alignment to rush into figure 2.

Level II

1. With your legs wide apart, loop two belts around the balls of your feet. Hold on so your arms are straight and your spine makes the smooth groove.
2. Slide your ischial bones just off the edge of the blanket.
3. Repeat Technique steps 1-4 and maintain the smooth groove with the legs and spine straight, as in figure 3.
4. *Only* if you can accomplish the above correctly, advance by bringing your legs hip-distance apart.
5. Keep your heels on the floor and grab the balls of the feet with your fingers for leverage to draw the body forward.
6. Yes, you will feel your spine more, but don't let the hips roll backward; keep working them forward, as in figure 4.

Tips

1. These sitting forward positions can be helpful only if you execute them at your own level of ability.
2. Remember, it's not what you do that counts; it's how well you are doing it that's important.
3. Periodically check your back with one hand to make sure you maintain your smooth groove (recessed spine).

Reference

Sitting Up on the Ischial Bones, and Sitting Forward Bend, section IV, chapter 3.

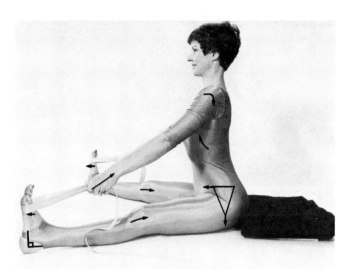

Figure 3

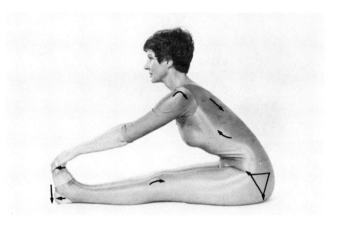

Figure 4
Level II
Sitting Forward Bend

2. Relaxation Technique

Most people consider relaxation as an "exercise" allotted to a specific time. Because Americans find it difficult to cause or create these time slots, they think they can't slow down, and tension builds. Actually, relaxation is a physical and mental letting go that should come naturally. It cannot be forced. Ideally, one should be able to maintain the letting go feeling at all times, for it is in this state that one's best work is done.

We recognize the problem of tension within ourselves and around us. The pace of life, current world conditions, constant movement through travel, and highly developed forms of entertainment, such as the television and the video boom, all tend to make our brain function at a speed sometimes too intense to endure for more than short spans.

The term tension is vague in meaning but its manifestations are easily recognized in symptoms that are all too familiar: inability to slow down, relax, or sleep; short attention spans; edgy nerves; and growing anxieties about everything and everyone. If these tensions are not dealt with, they can in time translate themselves into often-endured physical problems: headaches, colitis, ulcers, indigestion, malfunctioning gall bladders, high blood pressure (hypertension), heart trouble, poor circulation and, very possibly, even cancer. Some consider this lack of optimum health and well-being the price paid for progress in technology. Do not accept this assessment! Relaxation is within your control—treat it as your birthright.

Interestingly enough, you can "catch" tension from your neighbor in the same way as you can catch a cold when your physical resistance is inadequate. Conversely, you can avoid catching tension if your level of serenity is sufficiently high enough.

How can we integrate a more relaxed pace into our present way of living? First we have to learn to slow down from within. Strenuous emotional activity will speed up the heart, causing shallow breathing and weakening the oxygenation process until the whole system begins to feel the strain. This all happens because of a lack of harmony between our lifestyle and the basic rhythms of our breath, the misalignment of our bodies, and lack of self-confidence in our minds. To gain a total harmony, I have developed the Bodysense Method. If you have been following me through this book, you should be experiencing a new sense of balance in your body alignment, not just for an hour but day after day.

I have given you a thorough explanation of how to breathe correctly. Breathing is the most important ingredient in the

Bodysense Method. By learning to control your respiration, you can monitor and eventually control your feelings, emotions, and desires. The breathing process should set the pace of your physical activity. For example, when walking, you step in rhythm with your breath, as it leads you into nice, long, consistent strides. Maybe you don't walk this way; but I'm showing you that your breathing rhythm can be the fuel that ignites you instead of tensing you and blocking your natural harmony. Try applying the following breathing rhythm as you take long, swinging strides: Lift and open the chest on your *inhale* and try to get in three big steps, *hold* the breath on the next three steps, and *exhale* on the next five steps to completely empty out all the stale air. Your body now will be eager to breathe in again. With Bodysense awareness, you become more attuned to the rhythm of your breath. When you realize that you are in control, self-confidence and a sense of well-being can follow.

At first, you may think you are relaxing but watch your body closely. So many times, I've asked students to relax and they tell me with half-held breaths and tight jaws, they already are relaxed; but their bodies are reflecting that they are not. By breathing superficially, we suppress our feelings and create tension. When our breathing doesn't supply us with sufficient oxygen, our organs function at a slower rate, and our potential for sensory and emotional experience is reduced. This is a grim trap from which we seem to try to free ourselves—maybe we don't know we are prisoners. I hope through following the Bodysense Relaxation Technique, you will be able to experience the freedom of letting go so you can get to know the harmonious you.

When you practice the following relaxation techniques, don't force yourself to relax. I want you to connect with your own breathing rhythm that will allow you to let go. Instead of inhaling, make a big exhalation—have your breathing come in three steps: 1. *exhale* completely; 2. *hold* (pause) until you need air; and 3. *inhale* from deep inside the lungs. *Repeat* the rhythm. The hold creates a vacuum that compels the body to take a deeper, fuller, natural breath. It corresponds to the time necessary for the body to use the supply of oxygen brought in by the preceding breath. If you breathe this way, you will feel a deep, inner peace. The anxieties that have deformed your breath before, now give way to the authority of your body's natural breathing rhythm—You are in control!

Props

1. A carpeted floor.
2. Optional: a. a beach towel for under your thighs.
            b. a pillow for under your head so your neck will be aligned.
3. Tape recorder. I have written the Bodysense Relaxation Technique so you can read it slowly into a tape recorder. This will enable you to play it back for future, self-induced relaxation.

Body Placement

1. Lie down slowly on your carpet. To align your body, bend your knees; then take your hands and tuck your buttocks down and away from your sacrum. Slowly lower the legs. Check with your hands to make sure your pelvic triangle is level.

2. Bend your elbows and press them into the floor as you slightly raise your chest and elongate your spine. Rotate your shoulder blades down and inward. Lower the flat blades on the floor, feeling the chest free and open.

3. Zip up the back of your neck to elongate it and bring your head into balance and chin level with your forehead.

4. Extend your arms out from the sides so the armpits are open. Palms of your hands face upward.

Technique

1. Close your eyes and put all thoughts and distractions out of your mind Concentrate only on yourself and be aware of how you feel. Pretend you are taking a mental sunbath. * means *Wait* to listen and be attentive to yourself and the process.

2. Let your body gradually become limp and heavy; pretend you are slowly sinking into the floor.*

3. For the first round, the rhythm will be to breathe in deeply, tense up, and then let go suddenly with a concentrated sigh.*

4. Go down to the right foot; breathe in deeply as you tense it. Hold your breath, keep the foot tensed for a few seconds, then breathe out with a sigh. Release all the muscular contractions in the foot and feel it become heavy and sink into the floor.*

5. Keep the rest of the body loose as you tense each separate part. Now, inhale and tense the left foot. Hold the tension, exhale, and release.*

6. Breathe in deeply as you tense the right leg. (Keep the left leg loose.) Hold the tension and breath.* Release and exhale. Repeat by tensing the left leg. Hold* and let it go.*

7. Inhale, as you tense the buttocks and hold for a moment.* (Keep the rest of the body loose.) Release and exhale; feel yourself sinking into the floor.*

8. Take a nice, deep inhalation. Now, tense the chest and shoulders. Hold, breathe, and tense. (Keep your arms loose.)* Release the contraction in the chest and shoulders as you exhale.*

9. Go down to the right hand, as if to hold a great, big beach ball. Inhale, outstretch the fingers, and hold onto the ball, gripping tighter and tighter. The back of the hand stays on the floor. Now, exhale and let the ball go. * Imagine that it has bounced into the left hand. Inhale and outstretch those fingers. Hold onto the ball, gripping tighter.* Exhale and let it go.*

10. Inhale and elongate the neck. Exhale as you roll the head slowly to the right, taking time to lower it as far as it will

go.* Inhale slowly and roll it up to the center. Exhale, as you slowly roll it to the left. Hold* Wait for the count of two.* Inhale slowly and roll it back to the center.

11. Take a deep breath and tense all the facial muscles. Hold* and exhale, releasing (easing) the scalp, temple region, forehead, eyelids, and all the facial muscles.*

12. Feel your body let go,* as it sinks further into the floor.* Concentrate now on not moving your body so that you can relax even further from within. Next, you will center your attention on each individual part of the body as it is mentioned—relaxing without moving.

13. Continue throughout this portion to take deep, long, natural breaths. Going down your body, concentrate on the tips of your toes; relax them by withdrawing all activity from them. In the same way, relax the arches of the feet,* the heels,* the ankles,* the calves of the legs,* the knees,* and the thighs.* Your feet and legs are now completely relaxed and feel much lighter, as if they are floating on the floor.*

14. Now relax the buttocks,* hips,* abdomen,* and waist.* Relax all of them completely.

15. Going down to the lower lumbar region, relax one vertebra at a time, working up the spine.*****

16. When you reach the thoracic region, relax the rib cage. Your breath has slowed down now and is hardly noticeable. Let the feeling of relaxation gradually overtake the whole body.****

17. Going up the spine, relax the shoulder blades, come around front, and relax the chest. Just let those shoulders go and sink into the floor.*****

18. Going down now to the hands, feel the warmth and energy in the palms of the hands. Relax them* and also the wrists,* elbows,* upper arms,* those shoulders again,* and neck.* Since you are not holding the head up now, relax the neck completely. Notice how much lighter the head feels.******

19. Focus your attention now on relaxing the scalp,* temple region,* and forehead.* Ease them completely, removing any frown lines.***

20. Relax the eyelids,* cheekbones,* nose,* and lips.* Let your jaw drop* and part the lips.* Drop the tongue,* the jaw again,* and relax the throat.*****

21. Just let yourself go, sinking into the floor. Be aware of how quiet and still you can be.******

22. Finally, relax the mind by visualizing a peace-inducing scene. For example, a beautiful garden,* a deep blue sky,* with soft, white clouds drifting in the sky.* Hold this image for some time,**** then dismiss it. Now, imagine that you are a cloud.* You feel so light,* so relaxed,* just floating in the sky, passing other clouds, gently gliding along above green valleys,* forests, and a small lake. See the reflection of yourself.* How refreshing to be so gentle and airy,* so free,* and content.*******

23. Now, dismiss all thoughts from your mind. Allow it to become completely blank, as if you were sinking into oblivion, all peaceful and quiet.****

24. Remain in this state as long as you wish.********* Then ever so slowly, roll over on your left side, bending your knees to hip level. Take three breaths in this position; then return on your back. Awaken, by taking some deep breaths and stretching the fingers, arm, legs, and the whole spine. Let yourself yawn and continue stretching slowly. Roll up into a sitting position.

25. You have now experienced the completely relaxed state and can do so again by yourself, whenever you wish.

26. Remember, *you* control your body; do not let *it* control you.

Tips

1. Review Corrective Sleeping Habits for the Neck, section IV, chapter 6.

2. Do not fall asleep; that is not relaxation but a separate state.

3. Make sure you lie on a firm, flat surface. You might enjoy covering yourself with a big towel or blanket.

4. Take your shoes off and wear loose, comfortable clothing.

5. If you are going through the relaxation process and find some muscles tensing up on you, acknowledge it and go back down and relax them until they follow your desires. Remember, *you* control your body.

6. Do each holding position for at least five seconds.

7. Concentrate fully on each part of the body on which you are working. If other thoughts come in, dispassionately watch them wander past without trying to become involved.

8. Students who wear soft contact lenses should refrain from tensing the eyes. Hard lenses should be removed.

9. Perform the Bodysense Relaxation Technique whenever you are tired, angry, upset, and brain-fagged. It is not a waste of time. It works!

10. If you find you need relief and cannot relax, close your eyes and take a few deep rounds of the Complete Breath, section III, chapter 1. Tune into the letting-go feeling.

11. If you are still tense, try five rounds of Alternate Breathing, section III, chapter 1. Five good, concentrated rounds are as good as an hour of nap.

12. Relaxation should be practiced after each exercise session in order to fully assimilate the benefits.

13. It helps to feel like a sponge—porous and open everywhere. Inhale with your whole body, not just with your lungs. Visualize the lifegiving energy of the surrounding atmosphere, as it is being drawn in through all the limbs, providing the whole system with revitalizing power and rejuvenating every tissue of the body.

14. Relax periodically throughout the day, and you will double your efficiency and well-being. If you doubt me, try it and see!

15. Rhythmic breathing and relaxation exercises enable you to overcome muscular tension and mental strain. You can restore the normal working order of your entire system and the relaxation of your body and mind, which goes hand in hand with your health, youth, happiness, and a long life.

3. Daily Living Habits

Learn to live twenty-four hours a day with a straight, aligned spine. The following Daily Living Habits will supply you with the incorrect and correct positions of your everyday living habits. Regardless of whatever level of exercise you have reached, you should give great importance to how you perform the various activities of your life: standing, sleeping, sitting, driving, and working around the house and on the job. Executing these actions incorrectly can undo most of the therapeutic benefits that the Bodysense exercises offer.

So please take the following material seriously and put yourself in the corrected positions. You will be amazed at how good you will feel. You'll be free of tension and have more energy and strength.

CORRECTIVE SLEEPING HABITS

On the Back

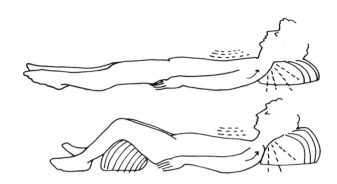

Pillow under shoulders.

Pillow under neck is too high.

Pillow under knees does not align the pelvic girdle.

INCORRECT

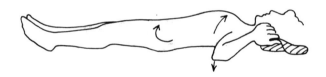

Slide buttocks downward.

Towel under the nape of your neck. See section IV, chapter 6.

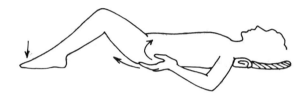

Press elbows down, pull pillow up under neck, lift and open chest, and lower onto flat shoulder blades.

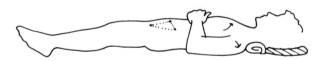

If pelvic triangle is level, you may rest.

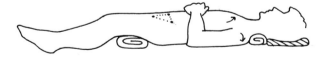

Use rolled beach towel to bring pubic bone up to level pelvic triangle.

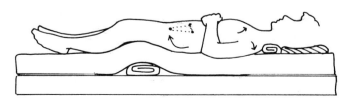

Place rolled beach towel under mattress.

CORRECT

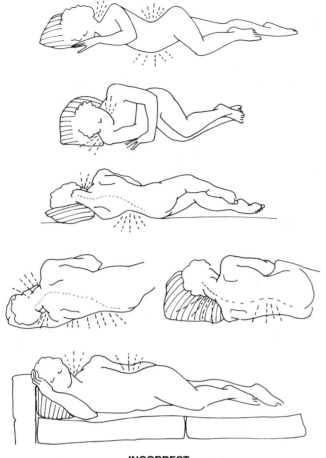

On the Side

It helps to place a small pillow between your knees.

The shoulders, hips, and knees are balanced on top of each other. See section IV, chapter 6.

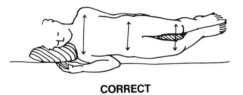

INCORRECT

CORRECT

On the Stomach

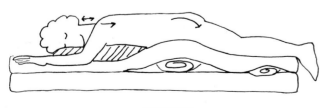

INCORRECT

Put a pillow under your head and chest and a rolled towel under the mattress at your hips and mid-shin of your legs the amount necessary to align your spine.

CORRECT

For Varicose Veins

Raising only the legs is not sufficient (for example, recliners), as the blood tends to get pooled in the pelvic veins.

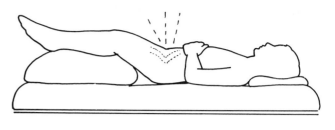

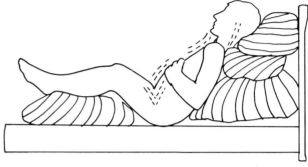

INCORRECT

Raise the foot of your bed or board under your mattress by four to six inches, so that both your legs and pelvis are elevated to further the downward flow of venous blood to the heart. Note the correct alignment.

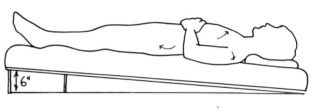

CORRECT

For Elevated Head

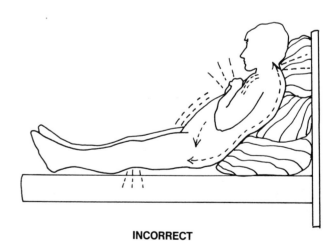

INCORRECT

- Hiatal Hernia
- Obesity
- Reflex Esophagitis
- Difficulty with Diaphragmatic Breathing
- Congenitive Heart Failure

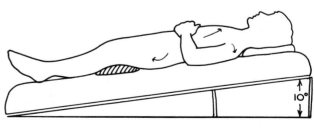

CORRECT

CORRECTIVE SITTING HABITS

At Home and Work

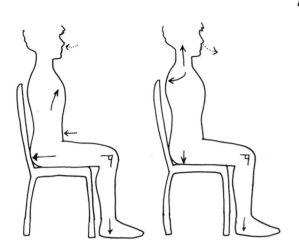

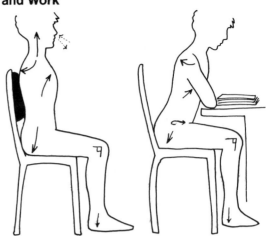

Slide your buttocks deep into chair.

Sit straight up on your ischial bones.

Use a pillow up behind your upper back for support.

Rotate your frontal hipbones forward to maintain alignment.

Sitting in a Standard Chair

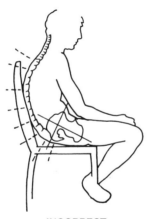

INCORRECT

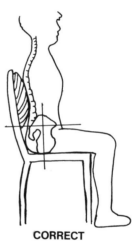

CORRECT

With Crossed Legs

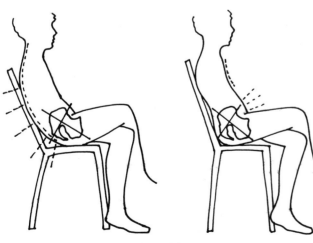

INCORRECT

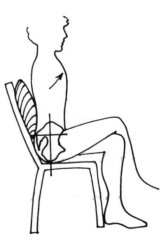

CORRECT

When the Chair is Too High

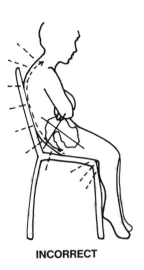

INCORRECT

Legs are too short for the chair.

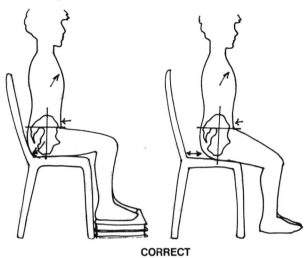

CORRECT

Raise your feet so the thighbones don't hang on the chair.

Sit toward the front of the seat so you don't need books.

At the Computer

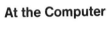

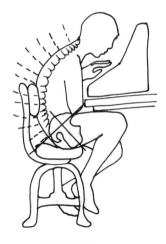

INCORRECT

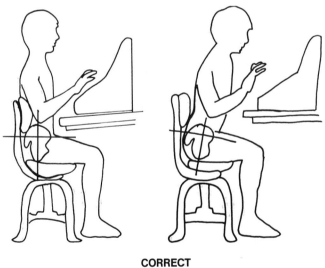

CORRECT

In a Recliner

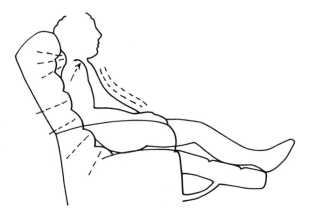

INCORRECT

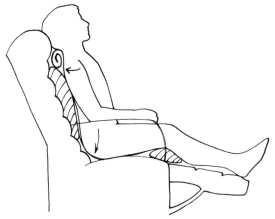

CORRECT

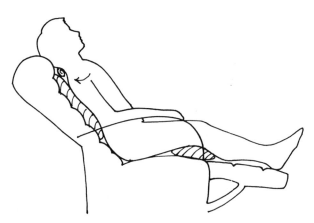

In a Kneeling Chair

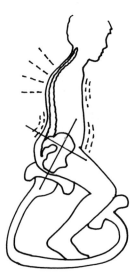

INCORRECT

Leaning too far forward and not using the abdominals for support.

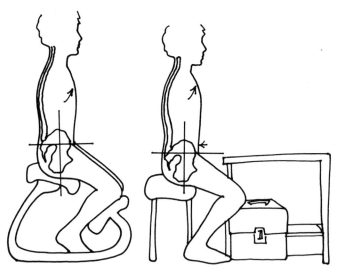

CORRECT

On the Toilet

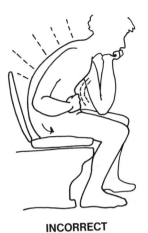

INCORRECT

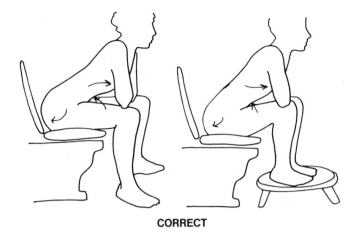

CORRECT

Raising the legs aids in rotating the hips.

In a Car

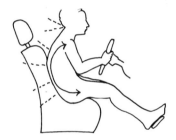
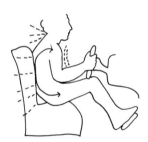
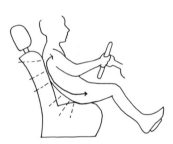
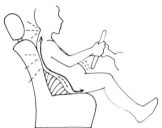

INCORRECT

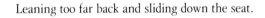

Seat is too far back, tilted, and soft.

Seat is upright but the body is not aligned.

Leaning too far back and sliding down the seat.

Pillow in the corner of seat is in an incorrect place.

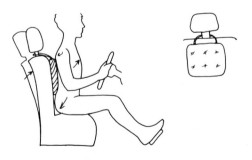

CORRECT

Rocking chair pillow tied to headrest.

Aim your buttocks deep into the back of the seat. Pull down on the steering wheel to elongate up out of your hips and open your chest. Place your flat shoulder blades against the pillow.

On an Exercise Bike

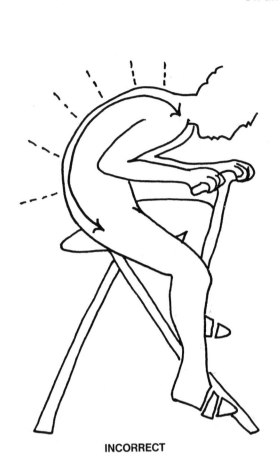

INCORRECT

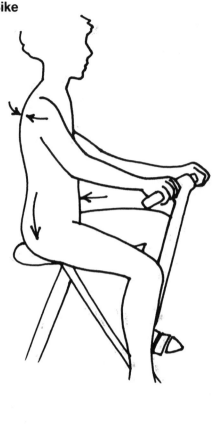

CORRECT

In an Airplane

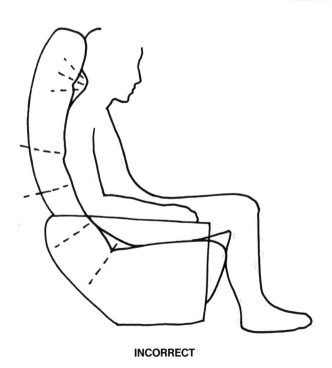

INCORRECT

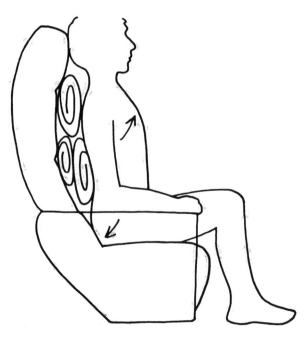

CORRECT

To Get Out of a Chair

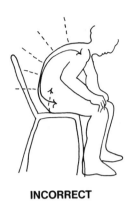

INCORRECT

Keep your spine straight. Don't round.

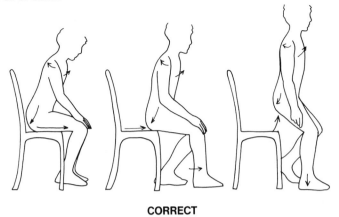

CORRECT

Step out and slide to the edge of the chair.

Use your legs, not your back, to lift off.

GUIDES TO EVERYDAY LIVING HABITS

Weight Bearing Standing

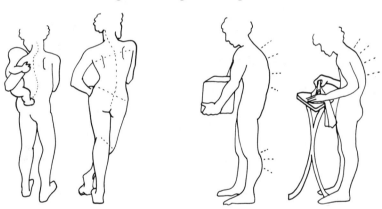

INCORRECT

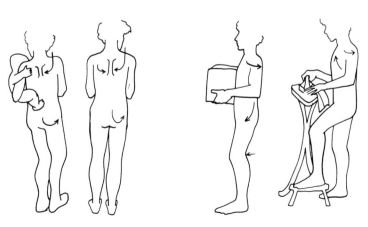

CORRECT

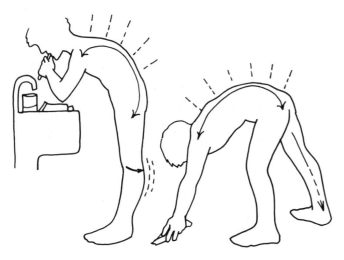

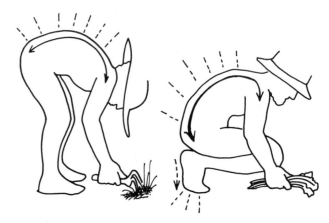

INCORRECT

"All I did was pick up a piece of paper."

INCORRECT

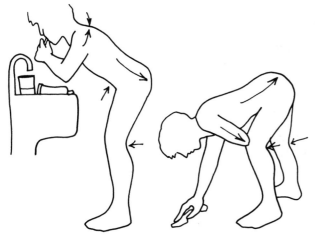

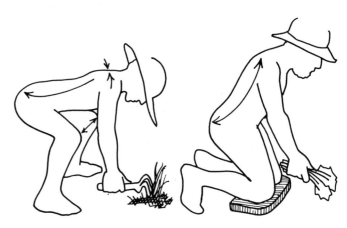

CORRECT

CORRECT

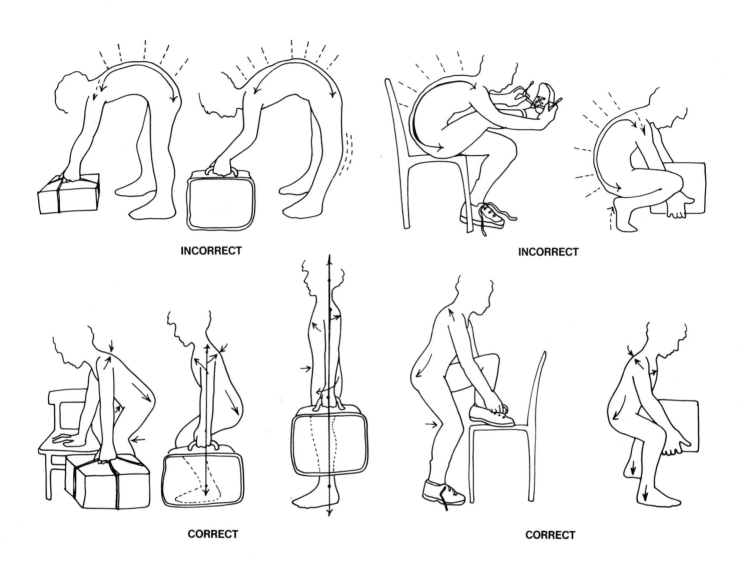

INCORRECT

INCORRECT

CORRECT

CORRECT

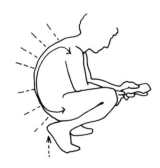

INCORRECT

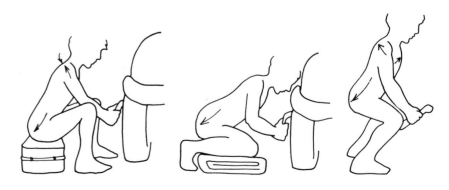

CORRECT

Push, Pull, and Shoveling

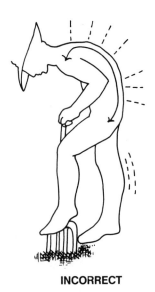

INCORRECT

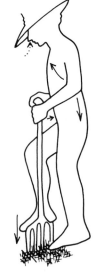

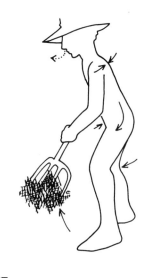

CORRECT

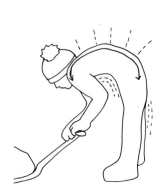

INCORRECT

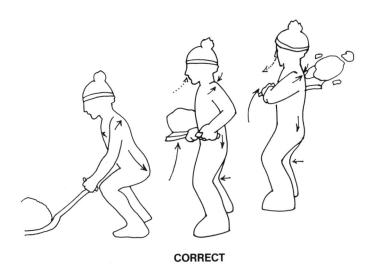

CORRECT

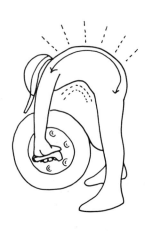

INCORRECT

CORRECT

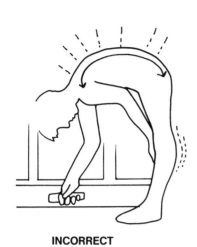

INCORRECT

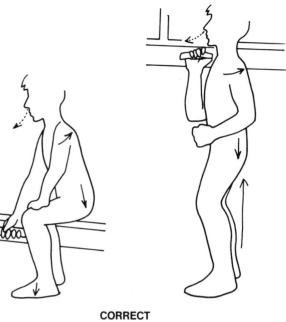

CORRECT

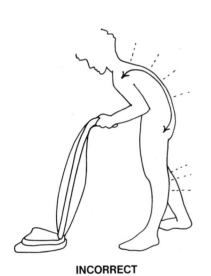

INCORRECT

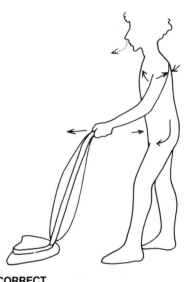

CORRECT

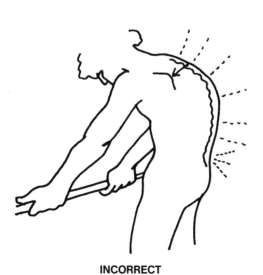

INCORRECT

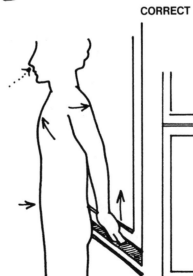

CORRECT

TIME SPECIFIC PROGRAMS

Five Minute

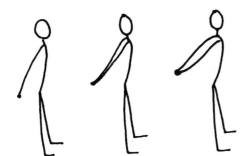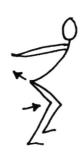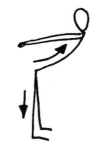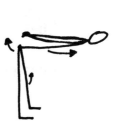

1. Chest Opener

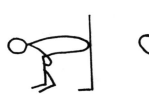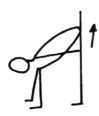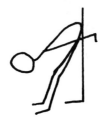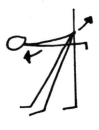

2. Hugging Hamstring Stretch

Ten Minute

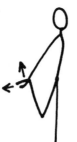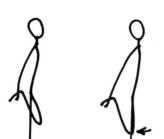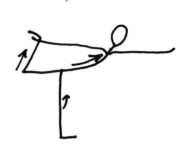

1. Quadricep Stretch

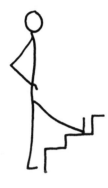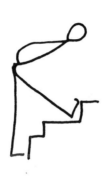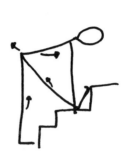

2. Standing Hamstring Stretch

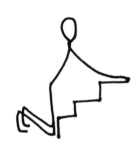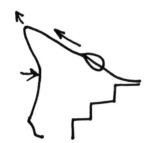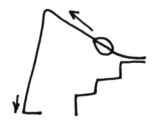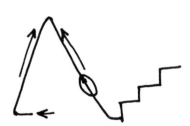

3. The Tent

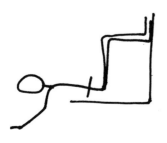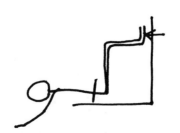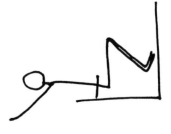

4. Sacrum Balance at Wall

Fifteen Minute

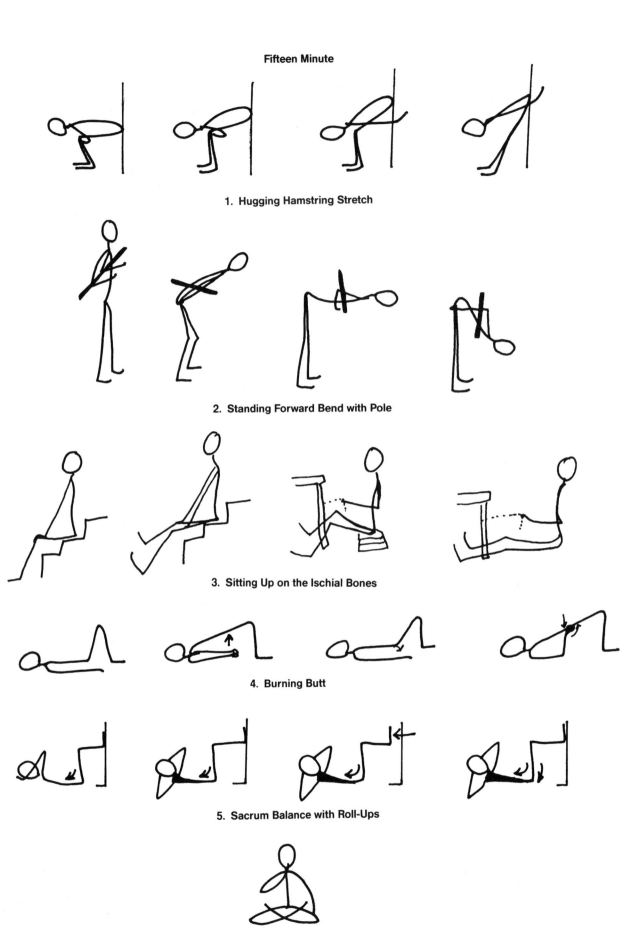

1. Hugging Hamstring Stretch

2. Standing Forward Bend with Pole

3. Sitting Up on the Ischial Bones

4. Burning Butt

5. Sacrum Balance with Roll-Ups

6. Alternate Breathing

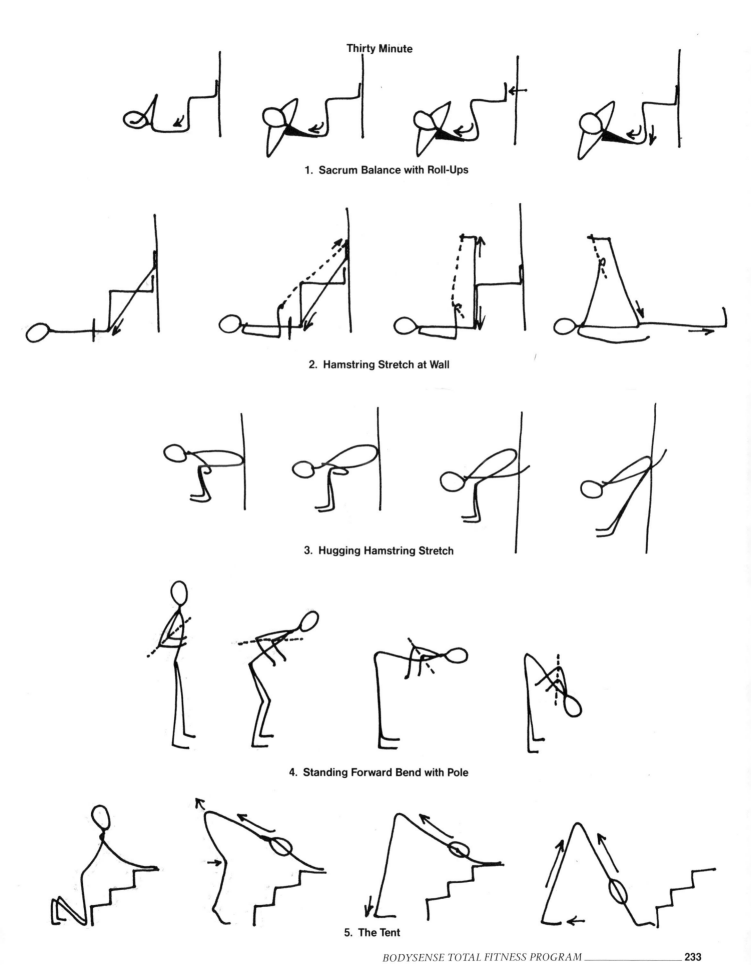

1. **Sacrum Balance with Roll-Ups**

2. **Hamstring Stretch at Wall**

3. **Hugging Hamstring Stretch**

4. **Standing Forward Bend with Pole**

5. **The Tent**

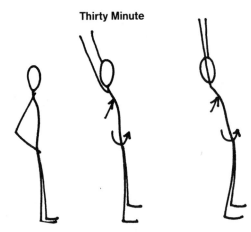

6. Elongated Back Strengthener

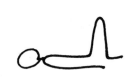

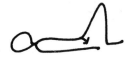
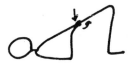

7. Burning Butt

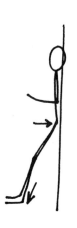
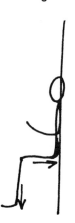
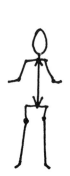

8. Strengthener for Hyperextended Knees—Phantom Chair

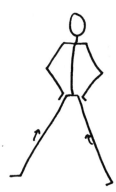
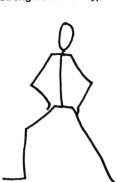
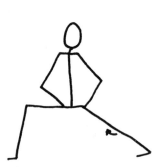

9. Front Facing Plunge

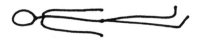

10. Bodysense Relaxation Technique

4. Bodysense and Beyond

Physical fitness is much more than physical activity; it includes psychological and emotional aspects as well. To keep ourselves truly fit on all levels requires a commitment to ourselves to become the best we can be. Bodysense is a viable vehicle to encourage that commitment. It issues a daily challenge to all of us, at any age, who have come to the realization that our bodies reflect ourselves and that we and our bodies can improve and keep on getting better throughout all stages of our lives.

As we come to know our bodies through the Bodysense Method, we can release the blocked energies of unexpressed emotions and limiting thoughts and free our minds and bodies from such unnecessary burdens. Then we can begin to picture the grace and elegance to which each of us is heir. We can feel and actually be younger than our years. We can enjoy an optimum measure of energy to live fully and respond totally to the daily challenges of life.

The body's potential responsiveness is limited by stiffness and lack of strength and endurance. The mind's responsiveness is limited by the way it thinks about people and things; it is often stuck in the past and sometimes in the future. Bodysense encourages us to be present in this moment—it is a living process of learning and exploring ourselves. Using it can provide us with a process for opening up and a chance to improve beyond our so-called physical and conceptual limits. We can transcend just functioning to using our bodies as a gateway for optimal conditioning.

A key to the process of opening up is what I call "playing the edge." The body's edge in Bodysense is the place just before pain, but is *not* the pain itself. Pain tells us where the limits of physical conditioning lie. Since the edge moves with subtle changes from day to day and from breath to breath, we need to be alert to know our condition for a certain moment. It is the *quality* of alertness as part of the meditative stage that is at the heart of Bodysense. For example, to attain proper alignment we should be aware of the requirements of a given posture, the feedback of our bodies, possible injury through carelessness, and the proper use of our breath. Once attentive, we can learn to become the passive observer of ourselves, midst both physical and mental activity. As we play the edge of what is physically possible, our edge moves. We have transformed what is possible. *We* have changed. There is more flexibility, more openness, and a corresponding increase of energy.

Another key in opening up is proper breathing. As we develop breathing techniques through Bodysense, the breath becomes a free-flowing bridge between our bodies and minds, which can further open pathways to a new sense of harmony. Bodysense is a total body program. It can enliven new nerve networks and muscle fibers that have lain dormant. Any new movement of one body part will be "lived" by the entire body. You can move with a unity born of the simultaneous combination of movements that flow together, rather than contradict, as so often happens in other exercise regimens.

The great danger in calisthenics is going on automatic so that the exercises become mechanical and stagnant, bringing with them dullness, fatigue, and an actual resistance to being fit. Bodysense replaces tedium with an active awareness that encourages us to go further because we can feel wondrous results in both our bodies and minds.

As we begin to recognize and respect our own physical rhythm, we discover new sensations and attune them with that rhythm. We learn not to rush, not to force, and not to sweat with overexertion, because working in a misdirected way blocks us from hearing our body's messages.

We often seek our sources—our reasons for having become what we are and our inner principles to become better than we are. Through understanding and working our bodies, we are able to align not only our physical well-being but our mental health as well. Bodysense work is subtle in its alignment, strong in its control, and precise in its execution. It is an invitation to know and love ourselves and our world. There is no such thing as a perfect exercise—it's the process that makes the difference.